ALOE FEROX
IN VIEW OF
AYURVEDA

A critical study of **ALOE FEROX** in
Ayurvedic perspective

DR. SHARDULI TERWADKAR

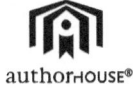

authorHOUSE®

AuthorHouse™ UK Ltd.
500 Avebury Boulevard
Central Milton Keynes, MK9 2BE
www.authorhouse.co.uk
Phone: 08001974150

First published by AuthorHouse 10/25/2011

ISBN: 978-1-4567-8786-8 (sc)

Any people depicted in stock imagery provided by Thinkstock are models,
and such images are being used for illustrative purposes only.
Certain stock imagery © Thinkstock.

This book is printed on acid-free paper.

PREFACE

It is an ancient practice to use herbs for wellbeing of mankind and it is ritualized in many ancient societies. It's amazing that we are still using this herbal knowledge but now with a new awareness.

With a surge of hundreds of books on herbs and uses of herbs in traditional and research point of view, people all around the globe are aware and well-informed with these ancient treasures of knowledge.

Students, Practitioners, Researchers and everybody interested in 'Herbology' are studying and using herbs in various ways.

Though there are many books introducing *Ayurveda* in scholarly ways, this book also introduces same theories in simplified way just to make readers familiar to the *Ayurvedic* terminology and basic theories of *Ayurveda* relevant to the subject.

While giving comparison between Aloe ferox and Aloe barbadensis, the latter is referred as *'Kumari'*. Though there are two species used as *Kumari*, Aloe vera and Aloe barbadensis, with reference to the original thesis, the latter one is described on the basis of availability of detailed references.

Focus of this book will be on introducing Aloe ferox, an Indigenous South African species of Aloes, with the application of *Ayurvedic* theories on its pharmacology.

We have tried to give a brief info about the *Ayurvedic* etiology and pharmacology regarding every medicinal use. *Ayurvedic* diagnosis is a complex method which considers all the details of your composition and checks every humor, tissue, system and even psychological factors while concluding about the diagnosis. This book will give basic logic behind the medicinal use mentioned. It will be every *Ayurvedic* Doctor's responsibility to apply this info with discretion according to patients' condition and other factors applicable while concluding about diagnosis, period of treatment and dosage.

We hope that this book will provide new topics to researchers in field of ethnobotany, ethnomedicine and herbology. It will stir brains of everybody who is interested in herbs and Alternative Medicinal Systems.

This knowledge definitely comes with a warning that medicinal uses suggested in this book should not be tried without experts' advice as herbs are potentially strong medicinal plants which can cause side effects if used irresponsibly.

On the same note, dosage is not clearly mentioned because it takes thorough checkup and discretion to decide a dose of any herb in *Ayurvedic* style of treatment. A tentative amount of dosage with fair idea about careful use and caution regarding treatments is given.

Wherever word 'cleansing' is used, it refers to *Ayurvedic* concept called '*Shodhan*' or '*Panchakarma*'. If Aloe ferox is used for cleansing, it should be used with discretion as per requirement of that case and should be preceded by *Snehan* (Internal and external usage of medicated oils to avoid adverse effects of cleansing) and *Svedan* (Fomentation of body to draw the toxins in to bowels).

As the description of all medicinal uses come with explanation of basic concepts and these concepts are again based on basic *Ayurvedic* Theories, repetition of few concepts and terms were unavoidable.

This book is written with main intention to provide a handbook for people interested in use of Aloe ferox to treat various medical conditions and that is why, every medicinal use comes with description of all theories related to that specific medicinal use, inspite of their repetition in the previous medicinal use.

Just open any page and find description about Aloe ferox and specific medicinal use you are looking for!

This research is open for any suggestions and views to take it further which will make this medicinal power more and more tangible in future.

We will certainly try to erase faults and improve this book in certain areas where improvement is possible. For all further updates and modifications on this book, please visit www.drsharduli.com.

For now, we are offering this humble effort to all of you out there striving to resolve mysteries of nature in all possible ways!

CONTENTS

CHAPTER I

A BRIEF INTRODUCTION TO *AYURVEDA*

Ayurveda - an ancient Indian Medicinal System

Ayurveda! Treasure of ancient medicinal knowledge! Foundation of many treatments, methods of treatments and techniques of modern medicine! A complete and organized system of medicinal science!

This introduction won't be enough if I want to introduce this ancient knowledge in scientific point of view. Let's go back to that very ancient time when we were nothing but just a part of living creatures on this Earth and were differentiated as a human.

Ancient quest for knowledge

Every ancient civilization has its unique ways to teach mankind how to live a fulfilling and happy life. This is because, man has always been curious to find out new ways to fulfill his needs.

When basic needs were fulfilled, his instinctive curiosity led him towards the other things surrounding him. This unending quest for knowledge turned out as several of sciences. Medical science is also one of those.

Man observed keenly the nature surrounding him and tried to imply things he learnt. He gave that knowledge to his successors which he got from the Mother Nature. As human beings, we have got a special gift from nature and that gift is - 'our highly developed brain'.

Our brain stores information in form of memory and makes it available in form of responses when it is required.

This knowledge is transferred to future generations and that is how humans were able to survive and even to shape their surroundings the way they wanted.

Cultural treasures of knowledge

All cultures have their own treasures of knowledge which originate and develop in that specific culture. That cultural pool of knowledge has a peculiar impression of geographical, geological and historical aspect of that specific culture.

It is also true for medical science.

Medical science shows various forms in various parts of the World. According to environmental factors and cultural forms, physical-mental-spiritual requirements of humans show variation. That is the reason why traditional forms of medical science shows some differences in different cultures.

It also gets restructured with time and becomes more and more applicable with time.

Cultural knowledge treasures those couldn't restructure themselves according to changing times, became neglected due to their old and unsuitable forms.

Very few ancient knowledge systems were able to survive and grow with time. One of those is *'Ayurveda'*!

Definition of Ayurveda

Word *'Ayurveda'* is combination of two words *'Ayu'* and *'Veda'*.

Ayu means life. *Ayu* is defined as a combination of body, senses, mind and spirit. This indicates that *Ayurveda* does not believe in cure of only 'body' but it is a complete regime for body, mind and spirit.

Veda means knowledge. It helps to take care of body, senses, mind and spirit.

Ayurveda is knowledge about living healthy and fulfilling life in all aspects. It is not just a traditional medicinal system but it is an ultimate guidance to live a quality life and to enjoy all aspects of our life.

Aim of Ayurveda

Ayurveda has a wide aspect of looking towards word 'Health'.

As we discussed before, *Ayurveda* deals with 'Life' which in *Ayurvedic* sense, is a combination of body, mind, spirit and senses. That is why, taking care of health in *Ayurvedic* sense, is taking care of mind, soul and senses along-with body.

As a complete science of life, it aims for taking care of healthy people which is preventive aspect of this science.

As a complete medicinal knowledge system, it has discussed about all the imbalances and manifestations of these imbalances in our body as diseases. In this part of *Ayurveda*, it guides the common people and practitioners to uproot the main cause of the disease or imbalance with the help of special diet, activity routine and *Ayurvedic* formulations.

3

Ayurveda doesn't stop with the only cure of problem but it also has strong prophylactic guidance for all kind of health problems which helps people to avoid recurrence of health problems.

As we discussed now, first aim of *Ayurveda* is to teach people how to maintain their health. It also explains why we should take care of our health.

According to Indian Philosophy, every human life has four main goals to be achieved, or in precise philosophical words, we are born with some divine intention to live our life fully with these four aspects. They are, *Dharma-Artha-Kama-Moksha*.

Dharma - As a human being, we represent this universe in a wide sense. We are not a mere living existence, but we are part of 'Universal Energy' and this awareness about our 'energy form' is called as 'Spiritual Awareness'.

This awareness or quest of mankind about knowing 'True nature of ourself', is explained in all civilizations in different ways.

Indian Philosophy also has explained about it and has guided about our duties as a human, as a part of society and as a subject of this world.

Word '*Dharma*' can be translated literally as 'religious duties' but more precisely it can be explained as a collective term for our family responsibilities, social responsibilities and religious duties which in all helps us to become more than 'a body'.

Artha - This word literally means 'earning'. As an intellectual and ambitious species on this Earth, man has always tried to earn more than food and shelter. Meaning of '*Artha*' encompasses many other things according to individual ambitions.

Generally this term includes all financial belongings and economical aspects like money, property etc.

We are always warned that we should strive for 'Artha' under the guidance of *Dharma* as extreme passion for 'Artha' can take us towards various crimes and most of all, towards unhappiness.

Kama – Literally this word means 'desire'. This word represents all human desires for various kinds of pleasures. Uncontrolled and wrong kinds of desires also lead to unhappiness and grief.

A person should try to fulfill all his desires under observance of 'Dharma', which helps us to live a successful life, in both aspects, material and spiritual.

Moksha – *Moksha* means salvation or union of human soul with supreme spirit which is named in different ways in different cultures.

All religions depict that this is the ultimate goal of a human being. Man has always been in search of this 'unknown yet tangible power' surrounding us. Though existence of soul is always questioned, all civilizations guide their people to look and grow themselves beyond mere physical, mental and emotional activities. Though it's not completely understood by everybody, we all can try to live with broad sense about life. While living a material life a person should always keep in mind that his actions should be thoughtful and responsible.

Ayurveda is praised in Indian Philosophy because it takes care of a 'body' which is a 'medium' to fulfill four main aspects of life.

Story of Ayurveda

Ayurveda is also born through the instinctive quest for knowledge. Word "*Ayurveda*" itself proves this.

Ayurveda means science of life and it is one of the most ancient sciences in the world.

5

Story of *Ayurveda* starts with the very first expression of knowledge in Indian Culture which is called as '*Veda*' which itself means sheer knowledge. Ancient Indian Culture and Hindu Religion is based on that knowledge given by *Veda*.

Archaeological references of ancient cities like *Mohanjodaro* and *Harrapa* show that Indian civilization which originated on the rich banks of rivers like *Sindhu* (Indus), *Ganga* (Ganges), *Saraswati*, was a completely autonomous and welldeveloped society with perfect city-planning having beautiful landscapes, majestic architecture, an efficient irrigation system and sewage-system. This well-organized society also had well-researched and well-documented sciences. Sciences like Astronomy, Astrology, Mathematics, Numerology etc are the boons given to us by this ancient civilization. Ancient scientist like *Aryabhatta, Kanaad* etc are wellknown for laying foundation of today's sciences like Astronomy, Physical chemistry and mathematics. This magnificent civilization faced many invasions and upheavals. Every time it sprang up from the destruction and not even fought the invaders also provided shelter for the visitors and refugees time to time. This open-minded civilization also shared its knowledge with many countries around the world since thousands of years. Many philosophers and scientists visited India time to time to get the knowledge of many ancient Indian Sciences. By preserving its own basic philosophy, this civilization also accepted new skills from these wise guests.

This whole story shows background of *Ayurveda*. *Ayurveda* is the medicinal knowledge of this rich civilization. Although these sciences were originated in ancient Indian civilization, like all great civilizations, these sciences were meant for wellbeing of mankind.

Vedic Philosophy is also one of those valuable gifts to mankind. *Vedas* are believed to be 'Divine Knowledge'. According to stories about origin of *Vedas, Lord Brahma,* The Creator of Universe, gave this knowledge to *Maharshis*, the great sages of India, who gave this knowledge to their students. This is the unique pattern of that ancient society which created a wonderful bond between *Guru* (Teacher) and *Shishya* (Student) and created a chain of knowledge from generations to generations. Originally it was learnt and inherited by word of mouth. After the invention of the art of scripture, it was stored in the form of scriptures on stones, wood and leaves. Then it was written on a special handmade papers and later on this skill developed as Scriptures in the form of books.

Vedic knowledge was differentiated in four parts; *'Rugveda', 'Yajurveda',' Saamaveda'* and *'Atharvaveda'*. All the four Vedas though focus on separate divisions of knowledge, mainly have spiritual aspect in their philosophy. Most of all the four *Vedas, Atharvaveda,* a form of *Veda* having information related to *Ayurveda,* mainly provides with spiritual solutions to all the health problems.

It is interesting to know how *Ayurveda* was developed or how it became identified separately. It is called as *'Ayurveda-avataran'*.

It is believed that *Ayurveda* appeared as divine words of wisdom in the form of division of *Atharvaveda* which was dealing with health related practices. That is why it is called as *'Upaveda'* of *'Atharvaveda'*.

There is another story which also emphasizes on divine origin of *Ayurveda.* When the Gods and the Devils were fighting for Immortality Potion called *Amrut; Lord Dhanvantari,* the God of *Ayurveda'* appeared with a pot of *Amrut.* This symbolizes importance of *Ayurveda* as a life saving knowledge since ancient times.

After appearance of *Ayurveda,* it was comprehended by Great Sage *Bhaaradwaj* who gave this divine knowledge to his students. Later on it was spread by these sages to the others.

If we look at these stories in different perspective, we understand that *Ayurveda* had a major role to play in history of Indian Culture. *Ayurvedic* experts were supposed to be Divine Souls as they were saviors. It was a fully developed and the most efficient Medical Science of that time in India.

Archaeological references show that ancient Universities of India called *Nalanda* and *Takshasheela* had thousands of books written by *Ayurvedic* Experts.

Samrat Ashok, who was one of the great emperors of India, was the first emperor who spread the principles of Buddhism and tried to re-establish peaceful society. This was the time when the magnificent universities like *Nalanda, Takshsheela* were teaching several of sciences to students from all over the world. Many students from other countries like Greece, China etc, came to India to learn subjects like Toxicology and some unique practices in *Ayurveda* like Cataract Surgery. References show that Cosmetic Surgery, Brain surgery, Prosthetics were done successfully in ancient *Ayurvedic* times which provide history of thousands of years to present day surgical knowledge. Maharshi Sushruta, an ancient *Ayurvedic* Guru, is called as 'Father of Surgery' in our modern surgical books.

In this Modern Age, new chapters in form of researches are joining this story and empowering this ancient knowledge with new aspects of studies.

Vedic root of Ayurveda

Archaeological references of *Ayurveda* date back approx. 5000 yrs B.C.

The scientific and systematic approach in organizing this knowledge is quite amazing.

Original references of *Ayurveda* seem to show the very first appearance in very knowledge system called Veda. Word '*Veda*' literally means knowledge. This knowledge dates back to almost 6000 yrs.

Veda was the ancient format of education that been passed on verbally from a generation to the next generation. Children used to get training about *Vedic Chanting* as part of basic education and later, due to vast span of this knowledge, everyone used to master himself in the branch related to their field of interest.

Veda was differentiated in four parts namely; '*Rugveda*',' *Yajurveda*',' *Saamaveda*' and '*Atharvaveda*', to make it easier to study and memorization of the hymns.

Every *Veda* deals with separate branches of knowledge.

Rugveda contains hymns praising knowledge and the Diviners.

Yajurveda is knowledge about self-defense which used to give knowledge and technical information about weapons and war skills.

Saamveda is the knowledge of arts especially 'Vocals' which is told as first ever expression of 'Art' in history of mankind. This is a complete science about Music.

Atharvaveda mainly deals with health problems which were mainly dealt with spiritual aspect in that time. That is why; rituals are main part of this *Veda*. Knowledge of *Ayurveda* emerged as side-trade of this main system. Impression of this original stream can be seen in original texts of *Ayurveda* in the form of some treatments given with rituals and hymns or *Shlokas*.

It is interesting to know how *Ayurveda* was developed or how it became identified separately. This process is called as '*Ayurveda-avataran*' (Appearance of *Ayurveda* on the Earth).

It is believed that *Ayurveda* appeared as divine words of wisdom in the form of division of *Atharvaveda* which was dealing with health related practices. That is why it is called as '*Upaveda*' of '*Atharvaveda*'. This branch of science must have emerged specially to deal with health problems of society, which can be seen in *Shlokas* that tell goals of *Ayurveda*.

It aims for two goals: Prevention of health of healthy people and complete cure of health problems of patients which also include prophylactic guidance.

9

It provides tailor-made health management to prevent health problems of individuals and to cure the diseases of individuals with natural medicines.

Later in *Upanishats* and *Brahmans*, references of this knowledge were again discussed with the philosophical point of view.

Basic Texts of Ayurveda

In *Vedic* times, *Ayurveda* was taught orally like other *Vedic* hymns.

After discovery of art of scripture, *Ayurvedic* Gurus documented this knowledge in the form of '*Samhitas*' or ancient texts. There are references found on leaves, bark and later on handmade papers.

Charak-samhita, Sushruta-samhita and *Ashtanga-sangraha* are called as '*Bruhattrayi*' or 'Trio of main texts'. There are three minor texts collectively called as '*Laghutrayi*' or 'Trio of minor texts'. They are as follows; *Madhav-nidan, Sharangdhar-samhita* and *Bhavprakash*.

Organised format of ancient Ayurveda

'*Asthanga*' literally means an entity with eight parts.

Ayurveda is a fully grown Traditional Medicinal Science which has eight different branches dealing with eight different subjects in Medicine. That is why it is also called as '*Ashtanga Ayurveda*'.

Eight branches of *Ayurveda* are as follows;

Kaya chikitsa- This is clinical medicine of *Ayurveda* which tells us about appearance of disease in six steps and how to control the disease on the specific step with the help of accurate diagnosis and treatment. As a complete health science of those times, it explains about etiological factors, pathological process, symptoms, signs, complications, prognosis, treatment and prophylactic care for diseases of all thirteen systems in body. *Maharshi Charak* is the 'Father' of this stream and *Maharshi Vagbhat* also dealt with this subject with vast research. These two *Gurus* created a long inheritance chain of students who also researched this subject thoroughly and revised the main texts.

Balaroga - This is 'pediatrics' of *Ayurveda* which tells us about taking care of children from newborns till 12 yrs. This branch explains about etiological factors, pathological process, symptoms, signs, complications, prognosis, treatment and prophylactic care for pediatric diseases and also for taking care of children from spirits.

Graha chikitsa - This branch deals with psychiatric disorders and also with disorders due to spiritual possessions. It also contains information about rituals and charms.

Urdhavanga chikitsa - This is the branch dealing with etiological factors, pathological process, symptoms, signs, complications, prognosis, treatment and prophylactic care for all the diseases of organs above the sternal notch (ENT)

Shalyachikitsa - This is the surgical branch of *Ayurveda* which explains about surgical tools and methods of surgery. Cataract surgery explained by surgical expert of *Ayurveda* named *Sushruta*, is still used for reference in Modern Ophthalmic surgeries. He was also the inventor of successful plastic surgeries, brain surgeries and prosthetics in those times. That is why; he is called as 'Father' of modern surgery.

Danshtra or Agadtantra - This is the Toxicology of *Ayurveda*. The Greeks were first to translate and introduce this *Ayurvedic* Toxicology to the west.

Jarachikitsa or Rasayan chikitsa- This is the branch dealing with geriatric disease management and rejuvenation therapies. All *Ayurvedic* texts have discussed this subject in detail as this is one of the popular branches of *Ayurveda* in all times. These texts have mentioned about miraculous effects of these treatments which was able to turn back the biological clock of body by decades.

Vajikaran Chikitsa- This is the branch dealing with etiological factors, pathological process, symptoms, signs, complications, prognosis, treatment and prophylactic care for sexual health problems and sexually transmitted diseases.

This is also one of the popular branches. It is actually more than the knowledge of aphrodisiacs because it was originally meant for treating sexual diseases and helping for reproduction of a healthy offspring.

One can see that *Ayurveda* has provided knowledge about all those subjects which a complete medicinal system should have.

Modern Syllabus of Ayurveda

Although *Ayurveda* is a complete science, as every science goes through, *Ayurvedic* medicinal system also has been researched deeply and constantly since thousands of years. Every generation of *Ayurvedic* experts has mentioned about their inferences through extensive research in all the ancient *Ayurvedic* texts like *Charaksamhita, Sushruta-samhita, Ashtaanga-sangraha* etc.

This continuous research has proved that *Ayurvedic* philosophy is a solid science in itself. That's the reason why, one can change the look of *Ayurveda* according to changed times, but always keep the original format same.

Now, in modern times, still *Ayurvedic* experts are busy in understanding the modern researches in medicines and *Ayurvedic* Doctors are keeping themselves well-informed.

Students of modern syllabus of *Ayurveda* have to learn all these subjects along with modern medicinal subjects too.

It not only helps them to get thorough knowledge of *Ayurvedic* medicine but also keeps them well-informed about modern medicinal practices and creates a wider conscious in their practice.

Learning and practicing *Ayurveda* makes all students and practitioners feel proud as they practice an ancient medicinal knowledge having a completely scientific approach and which is still helping the mankind in present times.

Isn't this feeling of every *Ayurvedic* Practitioner all around the world?

I know many people who want natural remedies with a scientific approach but are also curious about the logical explanation of that treatment.

It's every *Ayurvedic* practitioner's duty to introduce these people to *Ayurvedic* Philosophy in simple language to make them realize how these remedies work for them.

That will not only make them feel assured but they will also feel connected to our ancient quest which is nothing but 'profound knowledge of known and unknown world around them'.

CHAPTER 2

INTRODUCTION TO BASIC CONCEPTS OF AYURVEDA

Ayurveda aims for maintenance of health and if our health is disturbed then it helps our basic resistance by prescribing natural medicine with changes in diet and behavior.

I want to introduce basic theories of *Ayurveda* to make it simple to understand why your *Ayurvedic* Doctor prescribes you a certain diet, exercise and herbal combination.

Basic *Ayurvedic* Philosophy is based on these theories as follows:

1. Relation of man to the Universe
Man is mini-model of this universe which means we have everything in our body in a minute form what we have in this universe. That is why; our ultimate effort should be in tune with the Universe.

2. Material and Non-material make-up of the Universe
Ayurveda follows Indian Philosophy which says that this Universe is created with Material and Non-material things. Material substance is made of Five Primordial Substances called *Panchmahabhutas* (Earth, Water, Fire, Air and Space) and Non-material substance is made of

three omnisubstances called *Trigunas* (*Satva* or consciousness, *Rajas* or motion and *Tamas* or inertia).

3. Material and Non-material make-up of human being

Our body is also made of Five Basic Universal Elements called Earth, Water, Fire, Air and Space which can also be found in all living and non-living things on this Earth while our mental and emotional constitution is made of non-material substances called *Trigunas*. That is why; internal balance of our body can be changed by consumption of natural things.

4. Theory explaining about changes in body due to external things-

As we learnt before, *Ayurveda* believes that our body has all material and non-material substances just like all living and nonliving things around us.

It can also be said that we add substances having similar properties it accentuates the impact but if we add substances having opposite properties then it neutralizes or minimizes the impact of event in body ; this may be in the form of physiology or pathology.

5. Everything is medicine if used wisely

Nothing on this Earth is waste but on the contrary can be used as medicine if you have that special wisdom.

6. Three basic body humors (*Doshas*)

Our body has three basic humors called *Doshas* which are nothing but expression of *Panchmahabhootas* or Five Universal Elements in our body. They are *Vata*, *Pitta* and *Kapha*.

Vata is the energy in body which controls all the voluntary – involuntary movements of body and all the activities of body and mind. Utilization of air as our life source, function of respiration, maintenance of digestive system, circulation of nutrients, excretion of waste, functions of reproductive organ these all are the functions controlled by *Vata*. It correlates to functions of nervous system.

Pitta is the energy in body which helps in transformation of food into nutrition through the process of appetite-digestion-assimilation and absorption. Our appetite, digestion, quality of blood, intellect and health of skin and eyes depend on balance of *Pitta*. It correlates to digestive functions of body which also maintain micro digestion on the basic metabolism level.

Kapha is the energy in body which helps for binding and lubrication of our body which helps to build and repair our systems on cellular level. Protection of our digestive system by lubricating it, protection of our heart by maintaining its position and functions, protection of joints by lubrication, helping our tongue to decide the taste by producing saliva and protection of our nervous and mental activities by providing lubrication and nutrition to our brain.

7. Three basic mental humors (*ManasDoshas*)

Our body has three basic mental humors called *ManasDoshas*. They are *Satva*, *Rajas* and *Tamas* which are nothing but expression of *Triguna* or 'three types of omnisubstances' in our body.

Satva is pure state of our mind which gives complete realization or consciousness or pure knowledge.

Rajas provides us desire for activities or strive or motion or passion for something.

Tamas is inertia or ignorance which makes us flow with the desires and emotions and leads us to darkness.

8. Seven Basic Tissues (*Dhatus*)

Our body has 'seven basic tissues' called *Dhatus*. They are as follows:

Rasa – This is plasma or lymph which nourishes the body at cellular level.

Rakta – This is blood which provides life source to each cell which now we call as function of blood to provide the cells with oxygen and nutrients.

Mansa –This is musculature of our body that covers the skeleton and also performs the movements.

Meda – This is adipose tissue which lubricates and oils the cells and organs.

Asthi – This is bone tissue which provides support and protection to body.

Majja – This is marrow and nervous tissue which line the bones from inside and also carry the nervous functions of body.

Shukra – This is reproductive tissue which contains all the genetic data to propagate the life. This tissue in women is called as 'Artav' or 'StriShukra'.

Once these *Dhatus* are nourished they produce an essence of our health which is called as *Ojus* which is also called as 'aura' or 'energy'.

Ayurveda has explained that *Dhatus* produce certain by-products in their metabolism which are called as *UpaDhatus*.

They are again seven namely breastmilk (*Stanya*), menstrual blood (*Artav*), tendons (*Kandara*), vessels (*Sira*), oily substance in muscles (*Vasa*), skin (*Twacha*) and muscles (*Snayu*).

9. Three main types of excreta or *Trimalas*
Our body produces some waste in the process of metabolism which should be eliminated from body at its correct time. These excreta are mainly three:

Mala means feaces.

Mutra means urine.

Sweda means sweat.

Ayurveda recommends discrete study of *Trimalas*. They are important in our metabolism as their status shows us the status of our health.

There are some other byproducts called *Upamalas* which are secretions in nose and throat (*Mala-Kapha*), secretions in stomach and intestines (*MalaPitta*), excretions from organs, nails (*Nakha*), hair (*Kesha-smashru*) and sebum from skin.

10. Balance and relation of basic body components (*DoshaDhatuMala Siddhanta*)

All of us have all these basic components in our body as explained above but we have different permutations and combinations of those. We also have profound sense of the balance in body and mind on both levels; gross and subtle. This unique presence and balance of components makes our body different from others. Moreover our life depends on good balance of these basic components like three types of *Doshas*, seven types of *Dhatus* and three types of excreta.

When any component is disturbed it causes imbalance in organs or systems controlled by those components. Though all components are important in this complex mechanism, imbalance of *Doshas* is always the main cause of initiating imbalance of other factors or disease.

11. Theory explaining cause of imbalance in body components (*Samanya Vishesha Siddhanta*)

This theory says that if you consume any external ingredient like food, medicine and also follow behavioral pattern having similar qualities to that of any of *Doshas*, then it will increase the qualities of that specific *Dosha* in body. Vice versa; if you eat opposite quality food, medicine or follow behavioral routine, then it reduces qualities of that *Dosha*.

E.g. If you eat food which is dry and stale, it causes increase in activity of *Vata* which also include increasing dryness in body. This ultimately makes your skin look dry.

If you want your skin supple then you should consume food which is warm, juicy and fresh. This helps to regulate *Pitta* which performs function of maintenance of skin.

12. *Ayurvedic* Pathology - in short
Ayurveda believes that improper diet, behavior and external factors like micro or macro-organisms are the main cause of diseases.

Due to contact or consumption of above factors, *Doshas* get accumulated in excess or get aggravated or reduce in original quantity or also may get vitiated due to production of undigested, slimy and toxic by-product of impaired digestive function called *Aama*.

These disturbed or vitiated *Doshas* disturb the seven basic tissues, three basic excreta and sometimes spread even to the whole system related to that pathological process.

This is the *Ayurvedic* Pathology in short.

An *Ayurvedic* doctor has to go through all the subtypes of these *Doshas*, all seven basic tissues, seven byproducts of these basic tissues, all three basic excreta, all thirteen types of systems, al thirteen types of 'Digestive Fire' (macro and micro metabolism) of our body.

13. *Ayurvedic* Pharmacology - in short
As we learnt that *Ayurveda* believes that our body has all material and non-material substances as the living and nonliving things around us have.

We also learnt that adding substances having similar or different properties can change the process of pathology. It may be neutralizes or minimizes or maximizes the severity of pathology.

This theory in a different way says that material outside our body make changes inside our body either by increasing the power or decreasing the power of basic body humors. Substances having similar properties that of the body humors increase the power of those humors while substances having different or opposite properties that of the body humors decrease the power. That is how food and medicines affect our body and mind constitution. As food is also said to be nourishing our mind, it has emphasized a lot on selection of food as per constitution or to achieve certain changes in mind.

14. Body and mental constitution

Ayurveda believes that physical and mental constitution of our body is decided at the exact time of conception. Although seven basic constitutions are told, every individual has its own combination of factors those need to be decided by an expert. It has a unique way to decide basic body and mental constitution of a person which decides basic balance of humors in your body and mind. It is a thorough session in which *Ayurvedic* Doctors ask you questions and checks you from head to toe. Once your constitution is decided, it's easy to find out reasons behind the disturbances in body.

Ayurvedic treatment – Theories and techniques

Ayurvedic principles regarding treatment

Ayurveda believes that while treating a patient if you give medicines without proper cleansing of systems then it will be wasted. A very good example is given by *Ayurvedic Sanhitas* .They say that if you try to paint a very dirty cloth it won't get colored nicely. Our body also cannot absorb good medicine if systems are blocked with undigested nutrients especially *Aama* which is a sticky, slimy and obstructive product of undigested food due to low appetite and hampered digestion. This causes wastage of medicine, money and time.

Ayurveda recommends proper cleansing treatment which is called as *Shodhan Chikitsa*. There are five types of *Shodhan Chikitsa* which are also famous as 'PanchaKarma'.

They are *Snehan* (Oleation), *Svedan* (Fomentation), *Vaman* (Vomiting), *Virechan* (Purgation) and *Basti* (Enema).

Vaman is the best cleansing technique recommended for *KaphaDosha* while *Virechan* and *Basti* are recommended for *PittaDosha* and *VataDosha* respectively.

Before these three treatments a patient should go through proper course of *Snehan* (oleation) and *Svedan* (fomentation).

Oleation makes walls of systems smooth and supple while fomentation pulls out toxins and waste byproducts from channels and systems.

Then a proper cleansing treatment as per recommendation is done.

Then only recommended additional herbal treatment is given.

Basic things to check before deciding about treatment
Dooshya- Basic body components which get imbalanced or vitiated in pathological process are called as *Dooshya*. They are *SaptaDhatu* (seven types of basic tissues), *UpaDhatu* (byproducts of tissue metabolism), *Mala* (waste products) including main three excreta called *Trimalas* and micro-waste that is produced in microdigestion (*SookshmaMalas*).

Ayurvedic doctor should think about which *Dooshya* is imbalanced or vitiated.

Desh- As a science believing in relation between Universe and human body, *Ayurveda* also provides guidance about relation between geographical pattern and status of health or more specifically status of basic body components. These three geographical regions decided by *Ayurveda* are *Anoop, Jangal* and *Sadharan* which will be explained in detail later in this book.

Ayurvedic Doctor should think about Desh of the patient as imbalance of certain *Dosha* is more prevalent in certain *Desh*. Even this helps to decide dosage or '*Maatra*' of medicine. E.g. Patient living in *Jangal* or dry-hot-arid region should not be given strong medicines in comparatively large doses. I.e. medicines having *black pepper* or *mercury* and *sulphur* should be used only if required and in very very low dose.

Balam - This is body strength or muscle mass of patient.

Cleansing should be done very carefully in patients having very less muscle mass.

Kaala - Seasons of year are profoundly explained in *Ayurveda* and they are named as '*Rutu*'.

Six seasons according to *Ayurveda* are;

Vasant Rutu (spring), *Greeshma Rutu* (summer), *Varsha Rutu* (rainy season), *Sharad Rutu* (season after Rains has stopped and autumn is about to start), *Hemant Rutu* (autumn) and *Shishir Rutu* (winter).

In certain seasons, certain *Doshas* show certain conditions or status.

That is why it is very important to think about season to consider status of *Dosha*.

E.g. Medicines which can exaggerate actions of *VataDosha* should not be given in Rainy Season (*Varsha Rutu*) as *VataDosha* is naturally increased excessively in this season.

Agni - *Anala* or *Agni* means Fire. This is 'Digestive Fire'. Four types of 'Digestives Fire's are seen in four different constitutions.

Kapha constitution shows *Manda Agni* or low 'Digestive Fire'. It means low appetite and slow rate of digestion.

Pitta constitution shows *Teekshna* Agni or strong 'Digestive Fire'. It means they have very large appetite and strong digestive capacity.

Vata constitution shows *Visham* or irregular appetite with irregular and unpredictable digestive capacity.

23

People who have all Three *Doshas* in balance they show *Sama Agni*. It means average appetite which has average digestive power compared to other constitutions.

While giving medicines *Ayurvedic* doctor should decide about type of 'Digestive Fire' in patient. If a medicine having quality named *'Guru'* or 'heavy', is given in large quantity to a patient having low 'Digestive Fire', then he won't be able to digest that medicine completely and medicine will be waste. It will also confuse practitioner about expected results of treatment.

Prakruti - This is our physical and mental constitution which is explained in detail before.

Vayam - *Vayam* means age of patient. Dose of medicine needs to be changed according to age of patient.

Sattva - That is emotional or mental tolerance of patient. Some people don't like smell of alcohol or don't have much courage to face strong cleansing treatments like vomiting, purgation etc. In that case doctor should consider things tolerated by patient or only mild cleansing treatments or soothing treatments relatively.

Saatmya- We always have dietary and activity routine as per our geographical region and body needs. We are accustomed to certain types of foods and environment too. While consulting patients, *Ayurvedic* practitioners have to consider these habits of food, medicines and behavior of patients. In patients who eat Ginger in regular food, we have to consider some other plant as medicine or we have to give it in large amount to make it produce the desired effect in our body. Sometimes people have intolerance to certain medicines e.g. if patient is not used to medicines having strong smell, he may vomit the medicine.

Aahar- Practitioner also has to study food habits of patient. Medicines should be given according to food patterns of patient.

E.g patients who eat fish will appreciate medicines made of fish parts or combined with fish. Learning about food habits also helps a doctor to check nutritional level of patient.

There are many rules and regulations told by *Ayurveda* for practitioners.

Basic principle is taking out imbalanced and vitiated *Doshas* and maintaining their balance in body.

Main actions involved are Reduction of increased *Doshas* and Increasing *Doshas* which are very low in amount.

E.g. when main reason behind diseases is excessive oilyness or slimyness i.e. '*Snigdhata*', then *Rukshan* or dry treatment is used and vice versa.

When patient is having problems due to excessive '*Bruhan*' i.e. overnourishment due to consumption of rich food and lack of exercise, then the treatment producing lightness is used i.e. *Langhan*'.

Ayurvedic method of diagnosis
First step is deciding the constitution of patient.

Then diagnosis is made after 'head to toe checkup' of patient with thorough investigation of symptoms and sign.

In checkup, *Nadipariksha* or unique *Ayurveda* style checking of your pulse is one of the highlights of *Ayurveda*.

Ayurvedic Treatments
After careful checking and diagnosis about imbalance of humors and their spread in systems, treatment is decided.

Ayurveda offers wide range of treatments but your Doctor will decide the specific ones suitable for you. This is another peculiar feature of *Ayurveda*.

One for all doesn't work here!

There is a wide range of *Ayurvedic* Treatments but all work in three basic steps. Doctors decide if they want to go through all the steps for every patient or want to choose specific step with specific types of treatments for the patient.

These are basic steps:

Cleansing – If your body channels are clogged with toxins, all the efforts and medicines go waste. That is why, as per patient's strength and severity of diseases, a wide range of mild to strong cleansing treatments are given which are called as *Panchakarma*.

These are five main activities namely vomiting (*Vaman*), purgation (*Virechan*), medicated enemas and douche (*Basti*), instillation of medicated oils or powders in nose (*Nasya*) and removing impure blood (*Raktamokshan*).

Panchakarma are also recommended as prophylactic treatment to cleanse your body time to time to maintain your immunity and strength.

This is a thorough treatment which includes internal and external oiling of body, medicated steams, cleansing treatments and prophylactic routine with special diet and activities chart.

Digestion of *Aama* – In some patients if their 'Digestive Fire' is not working properly it produces an undigested, slimy, toxic, slug like material from food which clogs the channels and causes various diseases. This is called as *Aama*.

With the help of *Panchakarma* and some medicines, this *Aama* is removed and remaining is digested.

Alleviation or restoration of balance – According to *Ayurveda*, *Doshas* or three basic humors are the main cause of diseases in our body. They get accumulated or aggravated or reduced which causes imbalance in body. This leads to disturbed functions of *Dhatus* or 'Basic Tissues' and *Malas* or 'Basic Excreta' of our body. *Ayurvedic* Doctors remove the excessive or aggravated *Doshas* and disturbed *Dhatus* and *Malas* with the help of *Panchakarma* and give dietary routine and medicines to establish the balance.

Rejuvenation- This treatment is famous as regime which makes one look younger. In treatments it is used to erase the negative impact of disease from your body and set up a healthy constitution once again. It includes special diet, special behavior patterns and certain medicinal formulations.

This is an important part of treatment to strengthen the body resistance and to slow down the wear and tear of tissues. This, as a whole process, helps to decelerate the biological clock.

CHAPTER 3

INTRODUCTION TO AYURVEDIC PHARMACOLOGY

PROVIDED WITH GEOGRAPHICAL, GEOLOGICAL AND BOTANICAL KNOWLEDGE

Ayurvedic **Pharmacology (***Dravya-Guna-Vidnyan***)**

This is branch of *Ayurveda*, which deals with identification and pharmacognostic knowledge of medicinal plants which is used in treatments.

According to *Ayurveda*, every plant works due to active principles those are mentioned as '*Rasa – Vipak - Veerya* and *Gunas*'.

Rasa means Taste. This can be experienced directly or conclusions are taken about taste as per *Ayurvedic* principles told in *Ayurvedic* Pharmacology called as '*Dravya-Guna-Vidnyan*'.

Vipak means post digestive effect of plant.

Veerya means potency of plant.

Gunas means properties of plant.

Karma means pharmacological actions of the plant.

Concept of *Desh*

According to *Ayurveda*, *Desh* is a specific geographical pattern with specific soil pattern, climate and flora-fauna.

Ayurveda has divided geographical patterns into three types:

Jangal, Anoop and *Sadharan*

Jangal is a desert like or semidesert - like geographical pattern in which there is mostly arid land with less rainfall, less vegetation with mostly thorny, succulent plants, with dry, blowing winds.

Anoop is a coastal or highly humid forestation area like rain forests or beaches with hot and humid climate, with plenty of plants of all variety, variety of animals and birds, high rainfall, wide rivers or sea.

Sadharan is combination of these two types which is said to be excellent habitat for people.

New perspectives in research of *Ayurveda*:

According to my thesis, I have predicted *Rasa, Vipak, Veerya* of 33 medicinal plants of Southern Africa.

From these *Ayurvedic* predictions we can predict actions or medicinal properties of these medicinal plants which are called '*Karmas*'.

This study suggests more uses of various valuable Southern African Medicinal Plants and therefore increases usability of these plants. This will ensure a sustainable conservation of many of these precious plants.

Method of study:

An indigenous South African Medicinal Plants is compared with medicinal plant which is used in *Ayurvedic* treatments from ancient times.

Every botanical, morphological, pharmacological and ethnomedicinal aspect of these two plants is compared.

Taste (*Rasa*) and other qualities (*Veerya –Vipak – Gunas*) of indigenous South African Medicinal Plants are the major conclusions.

On the basis of these conclusions, pharmacological actions of the plant are explained.

Theoretical basis of the Study

*   *Ayurveda* is eternal and can be applied anywhere in this world. (*Ayurvedam Nityam*)

*   Everything in this Universe is made of Basic Five Universal Elements; Earth, Water, Fire, Air and Space (*Panchbhautic Siddhanta*)

*   Human existence is the miniature model of Universe and has all universal elements in his body. (*Pind-Brahmand Nyaya*)

*   *Ayurvedic* Pharmacology- All plants work due to qualities of plant namely Taste-Active energy etc. (*Dravya-Guna-Vidnyan*)

*   Everything in this universe is medicine including each and every plant. (*Aushadhitva* of all *Dravyas*)

*   Different theories to decide Taste of plant and other qualities. (*Rasoplabdhi Hetu*)

*   Continental Drift Theory - Drifting of Indian plate from Southern African plate may have some effect on plants of these two

countries. They may have similar qualities shown by Universal elements. (*Panchbhautic* qualities)

- Botanical Principles - Plants of same family and same genus show similar active principles.

- Pharmacognotic Study - Certain active principles show certain tastes (*Rasas*) in plants.

- Basic Five Universal Elements in a seed remain same everywhere. (*Panchbhautikatva of Beeja*)

- Taste etc qualities of plant change with environmental and geological changes. (Effect of *Desh* and *Bhumi* on *Rasadi GunaKarmas*)

- Intensity or strength of qualities (like taste) changes with change in environment of plant. (*TarTam Bhaav*)

CHAPTER 4

INTRODUCTION TO ALOE FEROX

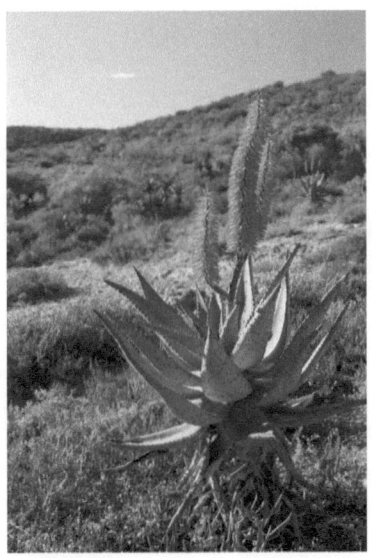

Botanical name: Aloe ferox

Family: Asphodelaceae (Previous name- Liliaceae)

Local names: Zulu, Xhosa, Sotho - Umhlaba
Afrikaans- Bitteraalwyn, Tapaalwyn
English- Bitter aloe, Red aloe

COMPARISON OF ALOE FEROX AND ALOE BARBADENSIS, MEDICINAL PLANTS OF SAME GENUS FROM INDIA AND SOUTH AFRICA

1. In botanical point of view, both plants are from same family i.e. Asphodelaceae and genus i.e. Aloe.

2. Both plants occur in variety of habitats but mostly require well drained soil, moderate water supply and areas with only moderate frosts but otherwise warm and dry climate. This type of geographical pattern is called as 'Sadharan Desh'.

3. Both plants show typical morphological characters of the genus, Aloe but have few differences. Aloe ferox is a robust plant compared to Kumari (Aloe vera) and shows flowers which are bigger in size showing dark red or orange colour. Aloe ferox do not show peculiar white spots on leaves.

4. Both plants show same active principle, Aloin, but percentage may vary because intensity of pharmacological action is different.

5. Exudates and leaf juice of both plants are used in medicines.

6. Aloe ferox do not have wide range of medicinal uses compared to *Kumari* (Aloe vera) and is mentioned as a toxic plant in South Africa.

7. Aloe-gel, slimy juice from leaves of both plants is used for skin and hair treatment.

8. Both plants are used as laxative in less dosage and purgative in large dose.

CHAPTER 6

PREDICTION OF PROPERTIES AND PHARMACOLOGICAL ACTIONS OF AN INDIGENOUS SOUTH AFRICAN MEDICINAL PLANT, ALOE FEROX

We can predict taste, active energy, post digestive effect, miscellaneous action, qualities of leaf juice, exudate and boiled / and dried forms of exudate or leaf juice of Aloe ferox on the basis of *Ayurvedic* theories.

Qualities of leaf juice

Taste- Bitter (*Tikta*), Sweet (*Madhur*)

Post digestive effect - Sweet (*Madhur*)

Active energy - Cold (*Sheeta*)

Qualities - Heavy (*Guru*), Oily (*Snigdha*), Slimy (*Picchila*)

Action on basic biological humors i.e. *Tridosha* –

Knowledge about action of this plant on three humors is very important. Once we know about the desired effects of this plant as treatment, we can combine it with other plants if we want some special balance in our treatment.

e.g. If we need a thorough cleansing effect by using Aloe Bitters without *Vata* aggravation, we can combine this plant with another material like oil, ghee or any other plant having antagonistic effect of *Vata* aggravation.

Lets have a keen look on actions of leaf juice of this plant on humors.

- **Cleansing of humors-**
  Humors get vitiated mainly due to *Aama* (undigested, cloggy and slimy product of action of low 'Digestive Fire') and macro and micro excreta like *Kleda* (excreta produced by *Kapha*).

  Due to laxative and purgative action, leaf juice helps to remove all excessive, aggravated or vitiated humors through the route of digestive system.

- **Alleviation of humors –**
  The traces of excessive, aggravated and vitiated humors can be treated by leaf juice as well.

  Due to its taste, post digestive effect and active energy, this plant has following actions on humors:

  Vata – Alleviates excessive and aggravated *Vata* due to 'Sweet Taste' and 'Post digestive effect' and all of its qualities.

  Pitta – Alleviates excessive and aggravated *Pitta* due to Taste, Post digestive effect and Active energy.

Kapha – Alleviates excessive and aggravated *Kapha* due to Bitter Taste.

- **Aggravation of humors –**
  Too much depletion of certain humor in body is also one of the causes of imbalances.

  Action of leaf juice of Aloe ferox as aggravator of humors is also helpful in such cases when certain humor gets too depleted in body.

  Let's have a look on action of leaf juice as aggravator of humors:

  Vata –In more dosage, it may cause *Vata* aggravation due to Bitter Taste and Active Energy. This action can be negligible due to Sweet Taste, Sweet Post digestive effect and qualities compared to similar action of bitters.

  Pitta – Leaf juice of this plant has one of the best sets of qualities as alleviator of *Pitta*. That is why, even in over dosage, it will never cause aggravation of *Pitta* humor.

  Kapha – Leaf juice of Aloe ferox can show action as *Kapha* aggravator as it has a set of qualities like 'Sweet Taste' (*Madhur Rasa*), 'Sweet post-digestive effect' (*Madhur Vipak*), 'Cold Active Energy' (*Sheeta Veerya*) and qualities (*Gunas*) like heavy, slimy and oily, which is the necessary set of qualities similar to *Kapha* humor. But this action will be possible only after very excessive dosage.

- Allover action can be correction of all three humors and it is safer as leaf juice has milder cleansing and alleviating effect than Bitters.

Local actions – Tonic for eyes (*Netrya*), treats nasal diseases (*Nasavikarnashak*), anti-inflammatory (*Shothhar*), painkiller (*Vedanasthapan*), removes pus from site and inhibits suppuration (*Pooyanashak*)

Internal actions – Eliminates faeces by breaking hard stools (*Bhedan*), removes excessive, aggravated or vitiated *KaphaPitta* by purgation (*Pittasarak*), laxative (*Anulomak*)

Qualities of dried form of exudate or leaf juice (*Saar*) or exudate (*Niryas*)

Taste – Bitter (*Tikta*)

Post digestive effect - Pungent (*Katu*)

Active energy - Hot (*Ushna*)

Qualities- Hot (*Ushna*), Strong (*Teekshna*), Light (*Laghu*), Dry (*Ruksha*)

Action on basic biological humors i.e. *Tridosha* –

- **Cleansing of humors** –
  Due to laxative and purgative action, Bitters of this plant help to remove all excessive, aggravated or vitiated humors through the route of digestive system. Action of Bitters is stronger than leaf juice due to its *Ushna-Teekshna* qualities which shows more dominance of Fire element.

- **Alleviation of humors** –
  The traces of excessive, aggravated and vitiated humors can be alleviated by Bitters as well.

  Due to its Taste, Post digestive effect and active energy, Bitters have following actions on humors:

  Vata –Alleviates excessive and aggravated *Vata* due to Active energy along with Hot property. In excess dosage, it may cause *Vata* aggravation due to Taste, Post digestive effect and properties like Strong, Dry and Light.

Pitta – Alleviates excessive and aggravated *Pitta* due to Bitter Taste, Post digestive effect, Active energy and properties like Hot and Strong.

Kapha – Alleviates excessive and aggravated *Kapha* due to all qualities like Taste, Post digestive effect, Active energy and all properties.

Overall action can be correction of imbalance of all three humors if used with discretion.

- **Aggravation of humors –**
  Action of Aloe ferox bitters as aggravator of humors should be studies carefully as it may jeopardize the desired effect in treatment if not used carefully.

  Lets have a look on action of Aloe ferox bitters as aggravator of humors:

  Vata –In more dosage, it may cause *Vata* aggravation due to Taste, Post digestive effect and properties like Strong, Dry and Light.

  Pitta – In more dosage, it may cause *Pitta* aggravation due to Taste, Post digestive effect and properties like Strong and Hot.

  Kapha – Aloe ferox bitters cannot show any action as *Kapha* aggravator as it hasn't the necessary set of qualities similar to *Kapha* humor.

Local Actions – Cleansing of wounds (*Vranashodhan*), healing of wounds (*Vranaropan*)

Internal Actions – Laxative (*Anulomak*), eliminates feaces by breaking hard stools (*Bhedan*)

On the basis of *Ayurvedic* interpretation of qualities of Aloe ferox explained above, we can use Aloe ferox instead of *Kumari* (Aloe vera) in various diseases.

We need to reduce the dosage as Aloe ferox shows more hot property (*Ushna Guna*) and strong property (*Teekshna Guna*) compared to *Kumari* (Aloe vera).

According to this study, leaf juice of Aloe ferox can be used as part of internal treatment in all types of rhinitis and complications of rhinitis explained in *Ayurveda*.

CHAPTER 7

PREDICTION OF NEW MEDICINAL USES OF ALOE FEROX

Aloe ferox as rejuvenating herb

Concept of rejuvenation according to *Ayurveda*

Ayurveda works on two fold goal; protection of health in healthy people and if these healthy people get some health problem, then *Ayurveda* intervenes with its knowledge about diet, activities and medicines.

Rejuvenation, according to *Ayurveda* is called as '*Rasayan*'.

Definition of '*Rasayan*' says that; this is the nourishing regime which re-establishes the health of all the seven types of basic tissues (*SaptaDhatu*) in our body. If a person has well-nourished tissues, then he also has well-functioning systems in his body, endurance and radiating energy. This is the sign of youth. That is why; this treatment was used to give the youth back to the person who desires for that.

Though this process needs a thorough cleansing of all body systems and channels, if patient is not strong enough to go through the deep cleansing, *Ayurvedic* practitioners recommend some preparations which act as mild cleansing and a good metabolism booster as well. This process acts in same way but affects on basic tissue levels systematically yet slowly. Once basic metabolism is improved, the balance between nourishment and excretion of waste or toxins gets established again. This helps for re-establishment of good quality and quantity of Basic Tissues. This allover imparts a good health, energy, immunity and youthful look to the person undergoing this treatment.

Pharmacological actions of Aloe ferox according to *Ayurveda*:

Aloe ferox shows all the qualities to decelerate the biological clock of our body.

We can use Aloe ferox as rejuvenating herb i.e. *Rasayan*, if we use various parts of this plant in combination.

Qualities and pharmacological actions endorsing rejuvenating action of this herb can be listed as follows:

I. Cleansing –

- **Purgation of accumulated excreta, parasites and toxins from body through bowels –** Due to purgative properties, Aloe Bitters can be used for thorough cleansing with proper care. This will help to remove all the excreta, toxins and parasites from bowels.

- **Cleansing of humors –** We can use mild laxative action of Aloe ferox for slow but constant removal of excessive, vitiated or *Aama*-mixed humors.

- **Removes *Aama* from body –** It can help to remove *Aama* produced due to improper diet and activity routines which affect all the 13 types of 'Digestive Fire' explained in *Ayurvedic* texts. *Aama* obstructs all the channels in body and interferes with normal functions of humors. When *Aama* gets mixed with humors, it causes wide range of symptoms, from bodyache - mild fever up to severe symptoms like failures of vital organs. This action of Aloe ferox will help to remove *Aama* and *Aama*-mixed humors from micro-channels in body due to its qualities.

2. Metabolism booster –
Taste (*Rasa*), Postdigestive effect (*Vipak*) and Active energy (*Veerya*) along with its properties (*Gunas*) can help as effective medicine on symptoms like low appetite, digestion trouble, mal-absorption and ultimately malnutrition occurring due to altered functions of 13 types of 'Digestive Fire' in body. Though there are 13 types, other 12 types are dependent on main entity which is *Jatharagni* or 'Digestive Fire' situated in stomach, duodenum and pancreatic area.

Normal functions of this type of 'Digestive Fire' depend on status of *Pitta* humor in body.

Aloe ferox helps to cleanse the micro and macro-channels in body, removes root cause of digestive trouble which can be excessive and impure *Pitta* as well as helps to restore the functions of 'Digestive Fire', which all over helps to improve the function of digestion in body.

3. Balancing of humors –
As we have seen, leaf juice can be used as best regime for balancing the humors in our body. If we are using Bitters in treatment, then it should be used in discretion as it may cause *Pitta* and *Vata* aggravation in overdosage.

4. Nourishment of *Dhatu* –
As a next step, leaf pulp or juice can be used as nourishment for *Dhatu*. All actions of this plant can help to improve absorption and assimilation of nutrients in all basic tissues in the order which ultimately helps to produce a healthy tissue mass allover in our body.

This helps to improve health of skin, hair, teeth which are the visible measures of one's age.

This action can help to produce a good amount of '*Oja*' i.e. energy which gives a healthy and beautiful glow to our body along with good resistance to diseases.

This action allover is nothing but action of rejuvenation.

5. Antiparasitic and antimicrobial action –
Aloe ferox can show action as anti-parasitic (*Krumighna*) and as anti-microbial which can be used to treat liver problems due to parasitic infestations or infections.

Methods of treatment:
We can use Cape aloe or yellowish leaf juice of Aloe ferox as cleansing treatment in low doses as first step for few days. We can use these bitters in a dosage of

After a good cleansing regime, when a person will feel lightness and cleanness in the body and when 'Digestive Fire' gets a good stimulation, we can start giving him pulp of leaf or fresh juice of pulp along with a very balanced diet as per *Ayurvedic* Texts.

Dosage should be minimum 10-15 ml everyday.

Caution:
Aloe ferox should be avoided in pregnant women as its use can cause abortions.

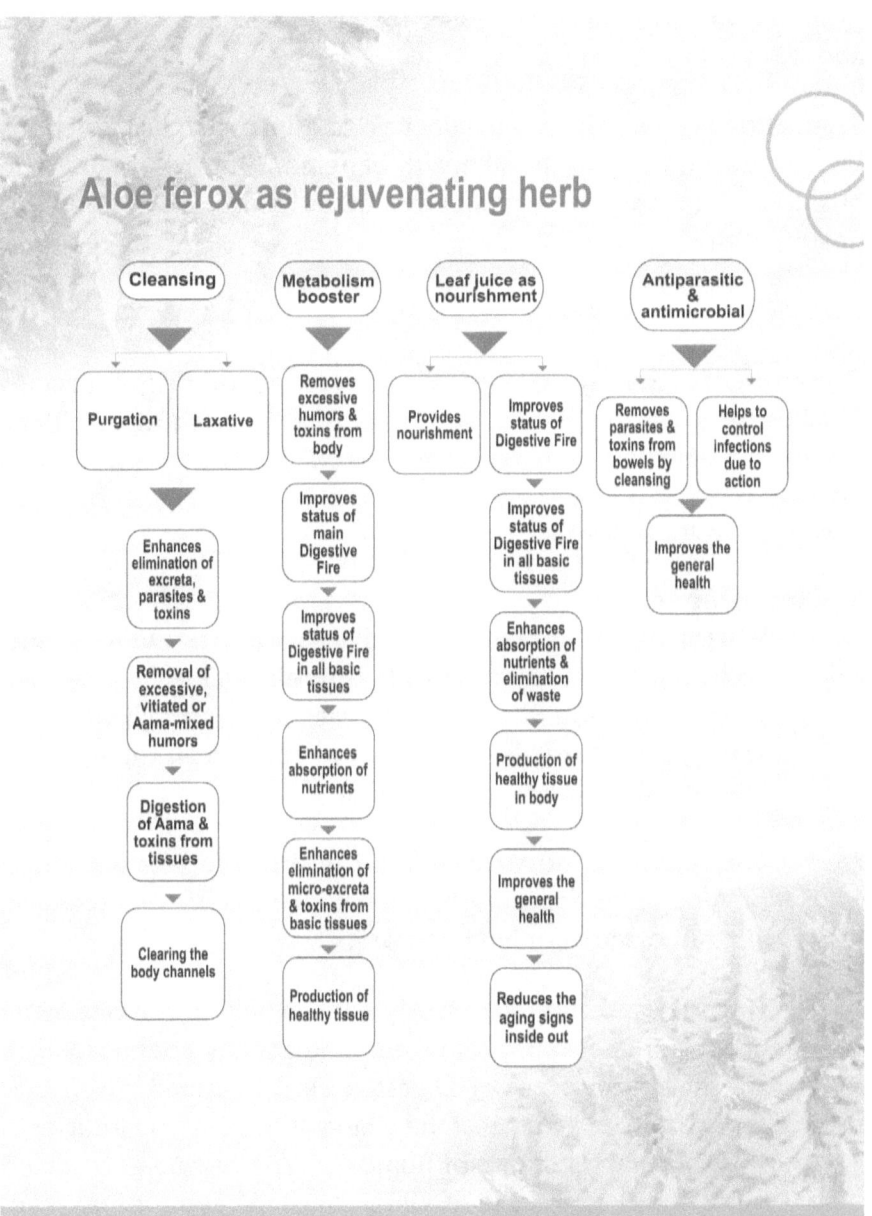

Aloe ferox as rejuvenating herb

Aloe ferox as an aphrodisiac

Aphrodisiac action according to *Ayurveda*
Ayurvedic definition of 'aphrodisiac' or '*Vajikaran*' has a broad aspect about reproductive function.

This action does not have only function to improve sexual functions but also encompasses general health of person, improvement in the quality and quantity of reproductive tissue which allover leads to healthy offspring.

Pharmacological actions of Aloe ferox according *Ayurveda*
Qualities and pharmacological actions of Aloe ferox show that it can work as an aphrodisiac in *Ayurvedic* aspect.

Let's list out its actions:

1. Cleansing –
- **Purgation of accumulated excreta, parasites and toxins from body through bowels** – Due to purgative properties, Aloe Bitters can be used for thorough cleansing with proper care. This will help to remove all the excreta, toxins and parasites from bowels.

- **Cleansing of humors** – We can use mild laxative action of Aloe ferox for slow but constant removal of excessive, vitiated or *Aama*-mixed humors.

- **Removes *Aama* from body** – It can help to remove *Aama* produced due to improper diet and activity routines which affect all the 13 types of 'Digestive Fire' explained in *Ayurvedic* texts. *Aama* obstructs all the channels in body and interferes with normal functions of humors. When *Aama* gets mixed with humors, it causes wide range of symptoms, from bodyache-mild fever up to severe symptoms like failures of vital organs. This action of Aloe ferox will help to remove

Aama and *Aama*-mixed humors from micro-channels in body due to its qualities.

2. Metabolism booster –

Taste (*Rasa*), Postdigestive effect (*Vipak*) and Active energy (*Veerya*) along with its properties (*Gunas*) can help as effective medicine on symptoms like low appetite, digestion trouble, mal-absorption and ultimately malnutrition occurring due to altered functions of 13 types of 'Digestive Fire'in body. Though there are 13 types, other 12 types are dependent on main entity which is Jatharagni or 'Digestive Fire' situated in stomach, duodenum and pancreatic area.

Normal functions of this type of 'Digestive Fire' depend on status of *Pitta* humor in body.

Aloe ferox helps to cleanse the micro and macro-channels in body, removes root cause of digestive trouble which can be excessive and impure *Pitta* as well as helps to restore the functions of Digestive Fires, which all over helps to improve the function of digestion in body.

3. Balancing of humors –

As we have seen, leaf juice can be used as best regime for balancing the humors in our body. If we are using Bitters in treatment, then it should be used in discretion as it may cause *Pitta* and *Vata* aggravation in overdosage.

4. Nourishment of *Dhatu* –

As a next step, Leaf pulp can be used as nourishment for *Dhatu*. All actions of this plant can help to improve absorption and assimilation of nutrients in all Seven Basic Tissues in the order which ultimately helps to nutrition of reproductive tissue (*ShukraDhatu*). This action allover is nothing but aphrodisiac action or *Vajikaran karma*.

According to *Ayurveda*, once quality of all the basic tissues of body and especially quality of those in reproductive system is improved; this helps to improve sexual function and promotes fertilization. This treatment can be used in the cases of infertility with discretion.

5. Antiparasitic and antimicrobial action –

Aloe ferox can show action as anti-parasitic (*Krumighna*) and as anti-microbial which can be used to treat problems due to parasitic infestations or infections.

6. Action of Aloe ferox in women as cleanser and hormone-regulator –

All the qualities of Aloe ferox show that if we use yellow exudates or Cape Aloe as cleanser in women who have irregularities of menses especially for them who don't have good flow of menses or have irregular menses. This plant will help to improve tone of uterine muscles and will help for cleansing.

If we use leaf pulp in same patients after thorough cleansing, that will help as a general health tonic and good nutritional supplement to improve quality of reproductive tissue.

Action of Aloe ferox as menstrual regulator proves the pharmacological action of this plant as herb which aligns hormonal axis in women, that's how Aloe species are used in *Ayurveda* since thousands of years.

Methods of treatment:

We can use Cape aloe or yellowish juice of leaf of Aloe ferox in very few doses for cleansing and as rejuvenation (*Rasayan*) or to assist rejuvenation (*Rasayan*).

With proper recommendation of diet, we can use Leaf juice of Aloe ferox as an aphrodisiac (*Vajikaran*).

It can be used as treatment on sexual malfunctions including infertility with discretion.

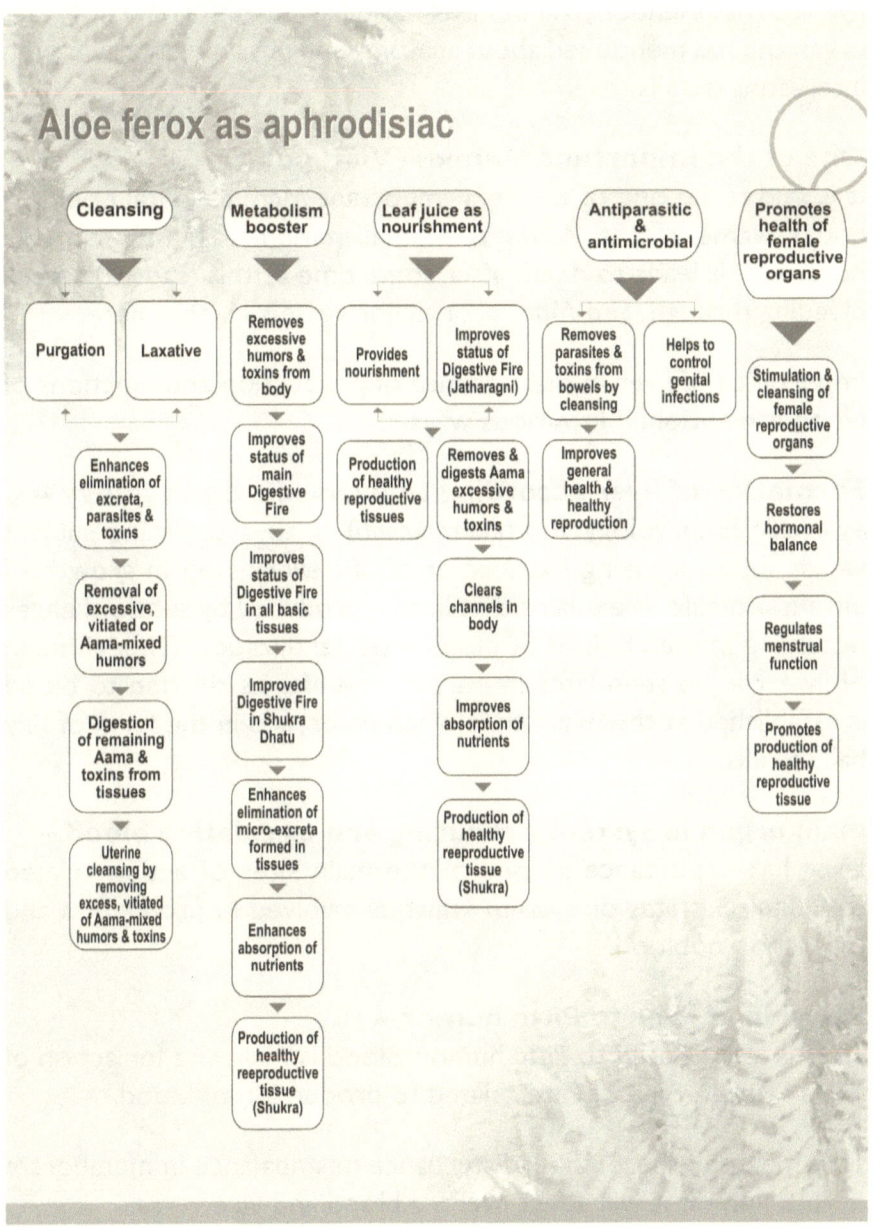

Aloe ferox as aphrodisiac

Aloe ferox as liver tonic

Ayurvedic description about liver

Ayurveda has mentioned about liver, called as *'Yakrut'*, as an important organ and has mentioned about anatomy and physiology of liver with interesting details.

One of the important *Marmas* (Vital point) –

It is said to be one of the very important *Marmas* (Vital points in body). Name of that *Marma* is *'BruhatiSiraMarma'*. If a person gets hurt here, it leads to death after some time as this leads to severe bleeding through *'Sira-Marma'* or major vessels located here.

Importance of liver in maintenance of production and functions of blood is mentioned in various ways.

Formation of liver according to *Ayurvedic* Embryology –

Ayurvedic Embryology (*Garbhaavakranti*) is an astonishing subject which shows amazing explanation about every step in growth of intrauterine life. It explains that liver is produced by subtle changes occurring in metabolism of blood after fertilization. Though form of liver can be seen later in intrauterine life, its relation to blood is established at the exact time when embryo is in the form of tiny ball of cells.

Main organ in system producing and circulating blood –

Liver has importance as one of the main sites of action related to *Raktavahasrotas* or system which is involved in production and circulation of blood.

Relation of liver to *Pitta* humor –

Liver is also related to *Pitta* humor. Blood is main site for action of *Ranjak Pitta*, a type of *Pitta* related to production of blood.

That means, if there is any disturbance or imbalance in metabolism of *Pitta* humor, it will affect liver via blood and vice versa.

Pitta humor is the main energy behind the food metabolism in body. If there is any imbalance in this humor, it causes malfunctioning of blood and liver. In the same way, if there is any imbalance or vitiation of blood or any liver problem, then it affects food metabolism of body.

Main site for *Raktadharakala* and *Purishadharakala* –
Acharya Sushruta has mentioned about a very special concept called '*Kala*'. *Kala* is a membrane or group of tissues covering the cavities in related organs to perform very special and subtle functions in metabolism of all factors forming body.

Liver has two important *Kalas*.

They are as follows;

Raktadharakala (Membrane or tissues covering the cavities in related organs which deal with production and function of blood); and

Purishadharakala (Membrane or tissues covering the cavities of organs which deal with absorption, assimilation of nutrients and formation of excreta)

That means liver play important role in absorption and assimilation of nutrients, production of blood, maintaining healthy quantity and functions of blood and last but important function is, separation of nutrients from excreta while maintaining quantity of body nutrients at healthy level.

It is simply amazing to read about all anatomical and physiological details of this important organ in such a systematic way and with a vivid description which dates back towards thousands of years.

Etiological factors and symptoms of liver imbalance according to *Ayurveda*
As *Ayurveda* considers liver as part of a delicate balance of humors, basic tissues and micro-metabolisms, imbalance of liver functions should be checked in all conditions in which all the systems are involved as mentioned above.

Impaired liver functions occur due to bad diet habits like eating food which is too much spicy or heat producing (*vidaahi*), toxic, too much secretion-producing food (*Abhishyandi*), stale food, indulgence in excessive alcohol etc and irresponsible, reckless lifestyle, addictions which aggravate or vitiate *Pitta*.

Factors which cause interference in functions of all types of 'Digestive Fire' are also responsible for imbalance in liver.

Other factors like infections and consumption of other toxic substances which can be explained as slow poisoning, are also etiological factors for symptoms of imbalance of liver functions.

Symptoms of malfunctioning of liver can be mild as loss of taste, loss of appetite, indigestion, flatulence and they can be severe as chronic constipation, pain, hepatomegaly, malnutrition, anemia, jaundice, ascitis and even abscess or growths. *Ayurvedic* guidance also tells us to check liver in skin diseases as imbalance of *Pitta* and blood also causes skin related symptoms as they affect liver.

There is a type of ascitis occurring due to liver imbalance which is called as '*Yakrutdallyodar*'.

One should treat these symptoms carefully after considering relation of liver to humors (*Dosha*), basic tissues (*Dhatu*) and excreta (*Trimala*) as well.

In conditions like aggravation or vitiation of *Pitta* humor by other excessive humors, toxins produced by microorganisms or *Aama* and symptoms of altered quality and quantity of blood (excluding internal or external blood loss), liver should be checked and treated along with as part of main treatment and prophylactic treatment.

Considering relation of *Pitta*, blood and liver according to *Ayurveda*, patients showing symptoms of altered functions of *Raktavahasrotas* also show symptoms of liver imbalance and should be treated with discretion and in line with any imbalance in liver.

Pharmacological actions of Aloe ferox according *Ayurveda*
We can use Aloe ferox as a liver tonic as per its qualities and pharmacological actions show.

Let's list out its actions as liver tonic:

I. Cleansing –

- **Purgation of accumulated excreta, parasites and toxins from body through bowels –** Due to purgative properties, Aloe Bitters can be used for thorough cleansing with proper care. This will help to remove all the excreta, toxins and parasites from bowels.

- **Cleansing of channels in liver directly –** Aloe ferox can help for cleansing the micro-channels and bile-ducts in liver. This can help for stimulation of bile production and regulating the normal flow. This can help to cure Jaundice and many other digestive problems originated due to improper functions of liver.

- **Imbalance of *Pitta* humor –** If liver trouble is due to aggravation or vitiation of *Pitta* humor, mild laxative properties of Aloe ferox can be used for a prolonged period. This action will also help for slow but constant removal of excessive, vitiated or *Aama*-mixed *Pitta* humor along with excreta and toxins produced due to imbalance in quantity and functions of *Pitta* humor. If there are symptoms due to vitiation of blood because of excessive, vitiated or *Aama*-mixed *Pitta*, then considering the relation of *Pitta* humor with blood and liver, we can use Aloe ferox for mild laxative action which helps in such interdependent pathological situations of liver, *Pitta* and blood.

- **Cleansing of blood –** We can use mild laxative action of Aloe ferox in liver troubles occurring due to malfunction or vitiation of blood. This action will help for slow but constant removal of excessive, vitiated or *Aama*-mixed humors especially *Pitta* from blood which will ultimately help to restore function of liver and again normalizes the function of digestion.

- **Removes *Aama* from body** – It can help in liver troubles occurring due to improper diet and activity routines which affect all the 13 types of 'Digestive Fire' explained in *Ayurvedic* texts, which cause production of *Aama* that obstructs all the channels in body and interferes with normal functions of humor. When *Aama* gets mixed with *Pitta* humor, it causes wide range of symptoms, from bodyache-mild fever up to severe symptoms like failures of vital organs. This action of Aloe ferox as metabolism booster will help to remove *Aama* and *Aama*-mixed *Pitta* from micro-channels in body due to its qualities.

2. Metabolism booster –

Taste (*Rasa*), Postdigestive effect (*Vipak*) and Active energy (*Veerya*) along with its properties (*Gunas*) can help as effective medicine on symptoms like low appetite, digestion trouble, mal-absorption and ultimately malnutrition occurring due to altered functions of 13 types of 'Digestive Fire' in body. Though there are 13 types, other 12 types are dependent on main entity which is *Jatharagni* or 'Digestive Fire' situated in stomach, duodenum and pancreatic area.

Normal functions of this type of 'Digestive Fire' depend on status of *Pitta* humor in body.

Aloe ferox helps to cleanse the micro and macro-channels in body, removes root cause of liver trouble which can be excessive and impure *Pitta* as well as helps to restore the functions of Digestive Fires, which all over helps to improve the function of digestion in body.

3. Balancing of humors –

As we have seen, leaf juice can be used as best regime for balancing the humors in our body. If we are using Bitters in treatment, then it should be used in discretion as it may cause *Pitta* and *Vata* aggravation in overdosage which is a big risk while treating liver diseases.

4. Nourishment of all seven types of basic tissues (*Dhatu*) –
In conditions showing malnourishment and loss of weight, we can use Aloe ferox as nutritional supplement for restoration of quantity and functions of all seven types of basic tissues (*Dhatu*). All actions of this plant can help to improve absorption and assimilation of nutrients in all basic tissues (*Dhatu*) in the order and will also help for healing of tissues of liver.

Nutritional qualities of leaf pulp of Aloe ferox can help directly as supplement.

5. Antiparasitic and antimicrobial action –
Aloe ferox can show action as anti-parasitic (*Krumighna*) and as anti-microbial which can be used to treat liver problems due to parasitic infestations or infections.

Methods of treatment:
We can use Aloe Bitters or Cape Aloe as purgative or thorough cleansing, with utmost care, in patients having severe symptoms and enough strength. In mild or chronic conditions and weak patients, Aloe Bitters can be used in low doses or leaf juice of Aloe ferox can be used for prolong period.

It can be used as supportive treatment or prophylactic for all severe or chronic symptoms and diseases like hepatomegaly, anemia, ascitis, jaundice, liver abscess or even to treat growths in liver.

In symptoms showing imbalance of blood due to *Pitta* or any other factor and malfunction of *Raktavahasrotas*, Aloe ferox can be used in any form to deal with the problem on root level, i.e. main site, which is liver.

Aloe bitters and leaf juice can be used in liver troubles due to parasitic infestations and infections. We can use leaf juice of Aloe ferox as supplement in all these conditions.

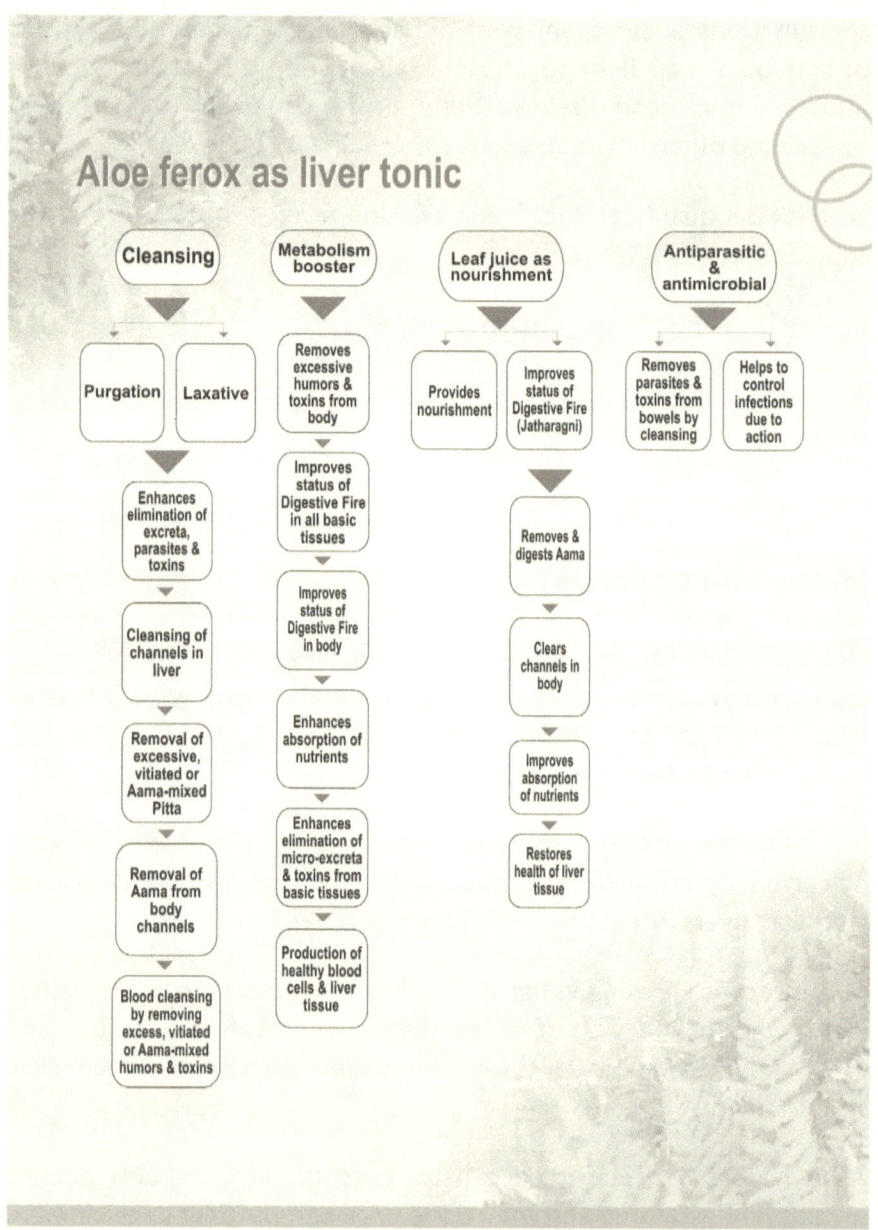

Aloe ferox for treating abscess

Ayurvedic concept of abscess:
Ancient *Ayurvedic* texts have mentioned in detail about various types of abscesses which are called as *'Vidradhi'*.

Maharshi Charak has explained about medicinal treatments of abscesses and also mentioned about a type called *'Vidradhika'* which occurs as a complication of diabetes (*Ayurveda* mentions this condition as a type of disease called *Prameha*) and is a type of abscesses related to diabetes (*Prameha Peedaka*).

Maharshi Sushruta, wellknown as surgical expert of *Ayurveda* and first ever plastic surgeon, has dedicated a complete chapter describing various etiological factors, symptoms, types and a wide range of surgical and medicinal treatments of abscesses.

Main two types of abscesses are explained on the basis of site of abscess:
- **External abscess (*Bahya-vidradhi*)** – This type of abscess is situated in skin, muscles and ligaments.

- **Internal abscess (*Antar-vidradhi*)** – This type of abscess is situated in cavities of organs or in abdominal region.

There are mainly six etiological factors listed:
- Improper diet and behavior which aggravates *Vata* humor,

- Improper diet and behavior which aggravates *Pitta* humor,

- Improper diet and behavior which aggravates *Kapha* humor,

- Improper diet and behavior which aggravates all three humors,

- External traumatic factors like bites, weapons or accidents,

- Factors producing toxins in blood

Though this problem is mainly treated surgically, *Ayurveda* explains various types of treatments to cure physiological factors causing abscesses.

Treatment of abscess is divided in following two stages:
- **Stage prior to softening of abscess (*Apakva-avastha*)** – Except in acute conditions, it is advised to apply external applications like packs (*Lepa*), Poultice (*Potis*) etc and to give *Ayurvedic* preparations as internal treatment to treat etiological factors and also as anti-inflammatory and analgesics.

- **Stage of softening of abscess (*Pakvavastha*)** – Once the abscesses starts softening and having pus formation, careful surgical drainage is advised. It should be done with extreme care and with appropriate prophylactic treatment.

Pharmacological actions of Aloe ferox according *Ayurveda*
We can use Aloe ferox for internal and topical treatment of abscess. The actions are explained below according to line of treatment recommended in *Ayurvedic* Texts i.e. cleansing, balancing of humors, nourishment of basic tissues etc.

Aloe ferox as internal treatment:
According to the qualities and pharmacological actions of Aloe ferox in *Ayurvedic* perspective, it can help in following steps as a treatment of abscess:

I. Cleansing –

- **Purgation of accumulated excreta, parasites and toxins from body through bowels –** Due to purgative properties, Aloe Bitters can be used for thorough cleansing with proper care. This will help to remove all the excreta, toxins and parasites from bowels. This action can be helpful in all types of abscesses except in internal abscesses or those closer to digestive system.

- **Cleansing of body channels –** Aloe ferox can help for cleansing the micro-channels in body. This action will help as general internal treatment in all types of abscesses except the conditions explained above.

- **Removal of excessive and *Aama*-mixed or toxin-mixed humors –** If there is tendency to have abscesses due to aggravation or vitiation of humors, mild laxative properties of Aloe ferox can be used for a prolonged period. This action will also help for slow but constant removal of excessive, vitiated or *Aama*-mixed humors along with excreta and toxins produced due to imbalance in quantity and functions of humors. If there are symptoms due to vitiation of blood because of excessive, vitiated or *Aama*-mixed humors especially *Pitta*, then considering the relation of *Pitta* humor with blood, we can use Aloe ferox for mild laxative action which will help in related types of abscesses. Again here we have to take care in case of internal abscesses or abscesses of digestive system.

- **Cleansing of blood –** We can use mild laxative action of Aloe ferox in abscesses occurring due to malfunction or vitiation of blood. This action will help for slow but constant removal of excessive, vitiated or *Aama*-mixed humors especially *Pitta* from blood which will ultimately help to cure abscesses and will restore functions of internal organs. Care must be taken in case of internal abscesses or abscesses of digestive system.

- **Removes *Aama* from body** – It can help in all types of abscesses occurring due to improper diet and activity routines which affect all the 13 types of 'Digestive Fire' explained in *Ayurvedic* texts, which cause production of *Aama* that obstructs all the channels in body and interferes with normal functions of humor. When *Aama* gets mixed with humors, it causes wide range of symptoms, from bodyache-mild fever up to severe symptoms like failures of vital organs. This action of Aloe ferox as metabolism booster will help to remove *Aama* and *Aama*-mixed humors from micro-channels in body due to its qualities.

2. Metabolism booster –

Taste (*Rasa*), Postdigestive effect (*Vipak*) and Active energy (*Veerya*) along with its properties (*Gunas*) can help as effective medicine on associated symptoms like low appetite, digestion trouble, mal-absorption and ultimately malnutrition occurring due to altered functions of 13 types of 'Digestive Fire' in body. Though there are 13 types, other 12 types are dependent on main entity which is *Jatharagni* or 'Digestive Fire' situated in stomach, duodenum and pancreatic area.

Normal functions of this type of 'Digestive Fire' depend on status of *Pitta* humor in body.

Aloe ferox helps to cleanse the micro and macro-channels in body, removes root cause of all types of abscesses (except one which is caused by external trauma) which can be excessive and impure humors. It can help to restore the functions of 'Digestive Fire' as well, which all over helps to improve the cellular level metabolism in body.

3. Balancing of humors –

As we have seen, leaf juice can be used as best regime for balancing the humors in our body. If we are using Bitters in treatment, then it should be used in discretion as it may cause *Pitta* and *Vata* aggravation in overdosage.

4. Nourishment of *Dhatu* –

In conditions showing malnourishment and loss of weight, we can use Aloe ferox as nutritional supplement for restoration of quantity and functions of all seven types of basic tissues (*Dhatu*). All actions of this plant can help to improve absorption and assimilation of nutrients in all *Dhatus* in the order and will also help for healing of abscesses and scars.

Nutritional qualities of leaf pulp of Aloe ferox can help directly as supplement.

5. Antiparasitic and antimicrobial action –

Aloe ferox can show action as anti-parasitic (*Krumighna*) and as anti-microbial which can be used to treat infected abscesses due to parasitic infestations or infections.

Aloe ferox as external treatment:

Aloe ferox can also help as a drawing agent having analgesic and anti-inflammatory effect. It can also help to draw local toxins and vitiated *Doshas* in the area of abscess and then helps it to get drained by itself by softening the skin.

Methods of treatment:

Ayurveda recommends that any type of abscess should be treated immediately by following line of treatment as explained above.

Aloe ferox can be used as part of main treatment or maintenance treatment or prophylactic treatment.

We need to supplement Aloe ferox with some herbs having predominantly anti-inflammatory and analgesic action throughout this treatment.

In case of internal abscesses or external abscesses near vital points (*Marmas*), careful surgical treatment should precede the internal treatment.

We can use Aloe ferox in packs or poultices as a drawing agent which will draw local toxins and vitiated humors in the area of abscess and then help it to get drained by itself by softening the skin. If it starts to soften and pus formation occurs then surgical drainage is recommended.

We can use leaf juice of Aloe ferox as dressing on the wound.

We can use Cape Aloe or boiled and dried leaf juice of Aloe ferox in very less dose for first step i.e. internal cleansing.

For external application, we can make a paste of those in water and can apply it on abscesses on limbs, back, neck and abdomen. When the abscess drains, we can use leaf juice of Aloe ferox as dressing on those wounds. This will act as antiseptic, anti-inflammatory, soothing and also as prophylactic treatment.

A person who has tendency to get abscesses frequently due to disturbed metabolism, stress, toxicity or due to chronic debilitating diseases like diabetes and even in AIDS patients ; we can use leaf Juice of Aloe ferox to improve their immunity to infections and to avoid tendency to get abscesses.

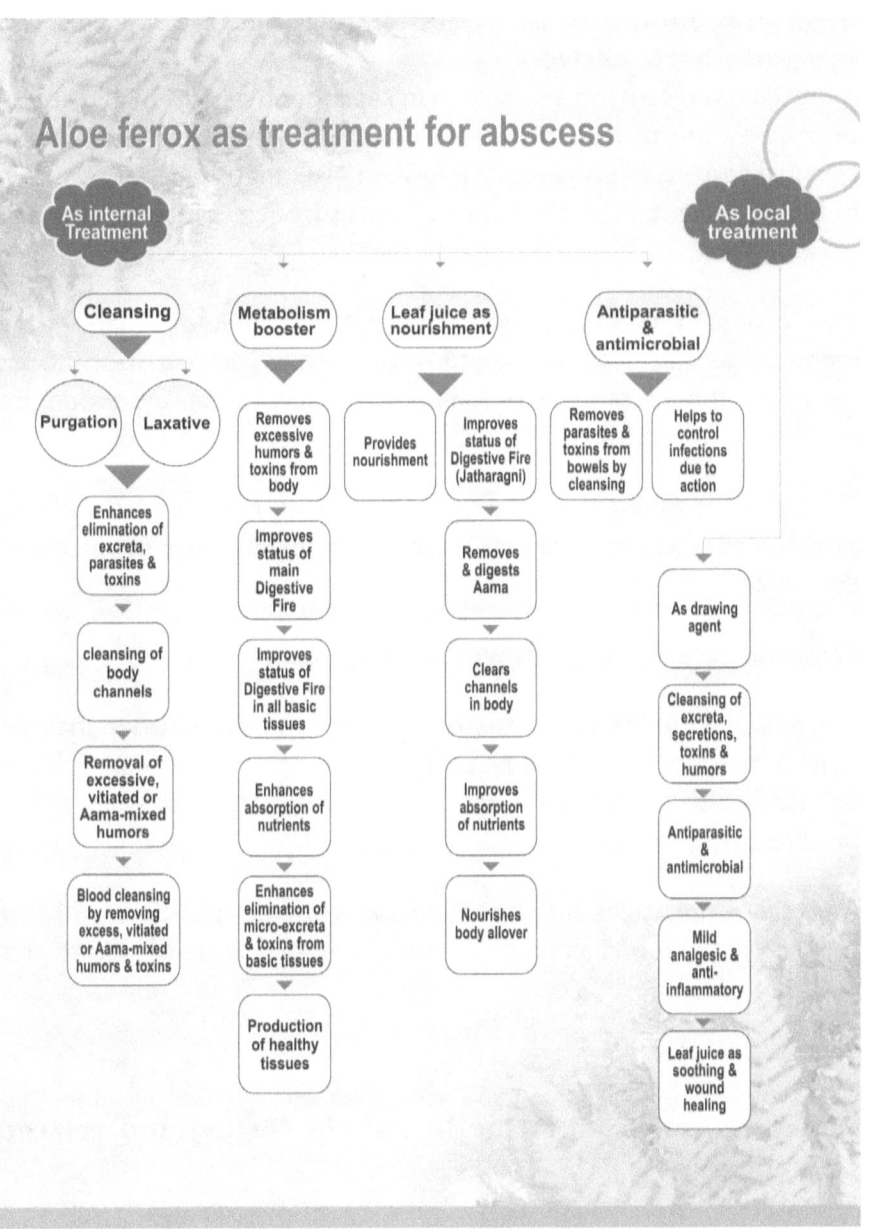

Aloe ferox as treatment for abscess

As internal Treatment

As local treatment

Cleansing

Metabolism booster

Leaf juice as nourishment

Antiparasitic & antimicrobial

Purgation

Laxative

Enhances elimination of excreta, parasites & toxins

cleansing of body channels

Removal of excessive, vitiated or Aama-mixed humors

Blood cleansing by removing excess, vitiated or Aama-mixed humors & toxins

Removes excessive humors & toxins from body

Improves status of main Digestive Fire

Improves status of Digestive Fire in all basic tissues

Enhances absorption of nutrients

Enhances elimination of micro-excreta & toxins from basic tissues

Production of healthy tissues

Provides nourishment

Improves status of Digestive Fire (Jatharagni)

Removes & digests Aama

Clears channels in body

Improves absorption of nutrients

Nourishes body allover

Removes parasites & toxins from bowels by cleansing

Helps to control infections due to action

As drawing agent

Cleansing of excreta, secretions, toxins & humors

Antiparasitic & antimicrobial

Mild analgesic & anti-inflammatory

Leaf juice as soothing & wound healing

Dr. Sharduli Terwadkar

Aloe ferox for correction of menstrual irregularities (Role as emmenagogue and uterine stimulant)

Brief introduction to female reproductive system in *Ayurvedic* perspective

Ayurveda has discussed about human reproductive system and action of procreation thoroughly in anatomical, physiological and even in spiritual aspect. Main texts of *Ayurveda* give anatomical description of female body and explain about various bones, joints, vessels and organs in it.

Milestones in life of a woman like menarche, pregnancy and menopause; are also explained with detailed information about care should be taken to maintain health in that time. Development of embryo into a full grown fetus is also described in detail.

Guidance for taking care in pregnancy is given month-wise and also includes precautions and treatments for delivery and problems in delivery.

Postnatal care is also given with neonatal care.

According to *Ayurveda*, status of reproductive system depends on diet, activities and heredity of parents and if a woman follows proper health guidance she can take care of herself at any stage of her life.

Ayurveda emphasizes on importance of woman in society which is only as 'female' but as a spiritual partner of a man to create this world in the divine vision.

Basic reproductive tissue in female (*Artav*) and related concepts –

Ayurveda thinks of reproductive system from the very early age, that is exact time of fertilization.

We need to understand three basic terms related to this system. Those terms are *'Artav'*, *'Stri-shukra'* and *'Raja'*.

Basic reproductive tissue is called as *'ShukraDhatu'* which is differentiated as *'Artav'* in females. This tissue is produced by involvement of 'Basic Five Universal Elements' which is mainly 'Fire Element' in female reproductive tissue. This tissue is nourished by prior tissues in the sequence of production i.e *'RasaDhatu'* (Liquid-tissue which nourishes whole body and is produced after action of 'Digestive Fire' on food) and *RaktaDhatu* (Blood).

These basic tissues get processed by specific metabolic factor called "Digestive Fire' of *ShukraDhatu'* (*Shukradhatvagni*) and produces *'Stri-shukra'* which keeps circulating in female body.

After a specific time (12 yrs according to *Ayurveda*), this *'Stri-shukra'* appears in the form of *'Artav* 'and *'Raja'*.

'Artav' is the *Ayurvedic* term for ovum. It is explained to be expelled from ovaries (*Andakosha* or *Pushpa*) every month and it unites with *Purush-shukra* to form embryo.

'Raja' or *'Artavsrava'* is the term used to explain menstrual flow which is also synonymously used with the term *'Artav'*.

Concept of *'Stri-shukra'* resembles hormone activity in female body.

There is another concept called *'Oja'* which is a factor produced last and is most important product of tissue metabolism which shows action that resembles the action called 'immunity' in our body. *Oja* is the byproduct of metabolism of reproductive tissue and it appears as a healthy glow all over our body. Some experts also refer this concept as hormonal secretions in our body that keep our body metabolism at its utmost function.

Signs and symptoms of healthy menstruation, which is called as *'Artavpravrutti'*, are given in detail. Etiological factors, pathological process, symptoms and treatments of abnormalities in menstruation and female reproductive system are also explained in *Ayurvedic* Texts under the title of *'Yoni-vyapat'*.

Description of ovaries and uterus according to Ayurveda:

Ayurvedic term for female reproductive system is *'Yoni'* and that is described to be having a shape of conch (*Shankha-akruti*). This term explains the screw- shaped gradually increasing space in the female reproductive system in the sequence i.e. external genital organs, vaginal tube and space in internal genital organs.

Ovaries are referred as *'Pushpa'* because of shape of the ovaries and fallopian tubes resemble a funnel-shaped flower, which is indicated by name.

Uterus is named as *'Garbhashaya'* that means space where a fetus (*Garbha*) rests in pregnancy. Detail anatomical and physiological explanation is given about this important organ which is one of the main sites of function in female reproductive system (*Artavavaha Srotas*).

These organs and related structures like bones, joints, vessels etc are also listed in Vital Points (*Marmas*) which emphasizes their importance in female body.

Concept of emmenagogue and uterine-stimulant according to Ayurveda:

Ayurveda mentions about certain abnormal conditions like less menstrual flow (*Alpartava*), abnormal menstrual flow with pain (*Kashtarva*) and heavy flow (*Atyartava*). These conditions are differentiated according to pathological factors involved and treatments are given accordingly.

Certain *Ayurvedic* preparations are used for local treatment and internal treatment as well which act as stimulants for uterus and ovaries. These preparations are called as *'Artavapravartak'* i.e. herb promoting and restoring normal menstrual cycle and *Garbhashayottejak* i.e. herb stimulating uterus to expel the menstrual blood and fetus where needed. Emmenagogues help to promote menstrual function by improving all over health of reproductive system while uterine-stimulants help to increase action of uterus to expel its products.

According to *Ayurveda*, due to improper diet and activities, humors get imbalanced and they affect the normal functions of 'Digestive Fire' in body.

Shukra (reproductive tissue i.e. ovum) is nourished last in sequential nourishment by *Rasa* and *RaktaDhatu*. If this sequence is disturbed, due to disturbance in 'Digestive Fire' of basic tissues, then it affects the normal growth of ovum. This affects normal menstrual function and fertility as well.

Sometimes normal menstrual cycle gets affected due to obstructions in macro and micro-channels in system due to various etiological factors explained in *Ayurveda*.

That is why an *'Ayurvedic* emmenagogue' is not a single action or action only focused on uterus; it is a combination of various actions which may take place all over the body but appear as uterine activity. It performs cleansing of body including reproductive system as well, metabolism boosting in all tissues including reproductive tissue, cleansing of blood to remove impure *Pitta*, unblocking of macro and micro-channels in body and reproductive system, improving activity of *Vata* and *Pitta* humor and also nourishment of reproductive organs, as required.

According to *Ayurveda*, *Vata* humor acting in pelvic region regulates the functions of uterus. When *Vata* humor is imbalanced then it disturbs the functions of uterus like changes in endometrium in menstrual cycle, holding foetus in pregnancy and expulsion of endometrial linings as menstrual flow while that of foetus and placenta in delivery.

Ayurvedic emmenagogues regulate these functions of *Vata* humor to promote normal menstrual flow while *Pitta* humor in blood regulates the quality and quantity of menstrual flow.

Ayurveda also considers activities of Five Universal Elements in this regard. Menstrual function is the action of Fire and Air Element. *Ayurvedic* emmenagogues are the combinations of medicines which balance and regulate these elemental actions.

Ayurvedic uterine-stimulant is again the action of *Vata* humor which also has contribution of Fire and Air Element.

Pharmacological actions of Aloe ferox according to *Ayurveda*:

Qualities and pharmacological actions of Aloe ferox shows that it can be used as emmenagogue and uterine-stimulant in *Ayurvedic* perspective.

Following is step by step introduction of actions of Aloe ferox in this regard;

Aloe ferox as internal treatment:

It can help in following steps as emmenagogue and uterine stimulant in irregular and obstructed menstrual flow along with other symptoms which indicate thorough internal cleansing:

1. Cleansing –
   * **Purgation of accumulated excreta, parasites and toxins from body through bowels –** Due to purgative properties, Aloe Bitters can be used for thorough cleansing with proper care. This will help to remove all the excreta, toxins and parasites from bowels. This action can be helpful in all types of diseases of female reproductive system (*Yonivyapat*) which need thorough internal cleansing of body through digestive system where it is applicable.

- **Cleansing of body channels** – Aloe ferox can help for cleansing the micro-channels in body. This action will help as general internal treatment in diseases which are caused by blockage of micro-channels (*Sookshma-srotas*) by micro-excreta (*Sookshma - mala*), *Aama* or conditions occurred due to other factors like parasites or microorganisms. This also helps free flow of *Vata* humor which also promotes its function.

- **Removal of excessive and *Aama*-mixed or toxin-mixed humors** – If condition occurs due to aggravation or vitiation of humors, mild laxative properties of Aloe ferox can be used for a prolonged period. This action will also help for slow but constant removal of excessive, vitiated or *Aama*-mixed humors along with excreta and toxins produced due to imbalance in quantity and functions of humors. Sometimes menstrual irregularities also show occasional overflows. These symptoms are due to vitiation of blood because of excessive, vitiated or *Aama*-mixed *Pitta*, e.g. in conditions like *Atyartava, Adhoga RaktaPitta*, then considering the relation of *Pitta* humor with blood, we can use Aloe ferox for mild laxative action which will help in all applicable conditions.

- **Cleansing of blood** – We can use mild laxative action of Aloe ferox in menstrual irregularities occurring due to malfunction or vitiation of blood. This action will help for slow but constant removal of excessive, vitiated or *Aama*-mixed humors especially *Pitta* from blood which will ultimately help to remove root-cause.

- **Removes *Aama* from body** – It can help in all types of conditions occurring due to improper diet and activity routines which affect all the 13 types of 'Digestive Fire' explained in *Ayurvedic* texts, which cause production of *Aama* that obstructs all the channels in body and interferes with normal functions of humor. When *Aama* gets mixed with humors, it obstructs the nutrition of basic tissues which produces weak or abnormal tissues. In relation with reproductive system, this can cause abnormal production of *Artav* which causes wide range of symptoms, from general symptoms like body ache-mild fever up to severe symptoms like abnormal menstrual functions and infertility. This action of Aloe ferox, as metabolism booster, will help to remove *Aama* and *Aama*-mixed humors from micro-channels in systems due to its qualities.

2. Metabolism booster –

Taste (*Rasa*), Post-digestive effect (*Vipak*) and Active energy (*Veerya*) along with its properties (*Gunas*) can help as effective medicine on associated symptoms like low appetite, digestion trouble, mal-absorption and ultimately malnutrition occurring due to altered functions of 13 types of 'Digestive Fire' in body. Though there are 13 types, other 12 types are dependent on main entity which is *Jatharagni* or 'Digestive Fire' situated in stomach, duodenum and pancreatic area.

Normal functions of this type of 'Digestive Fire' depend mainly on status of *Pitta* humor in body.

Aloe ferox helps to cleanse the micro and macro-channels in body, removes root cause of menstrual irregularities which can be excessive and impure humors. It can help to restore the functions of 'Digestive Fire' as well, which all over helps to improve the cellular level metabolism in women.

3. Nourishment of *Dhatu* –

In conditions showing malnourishment and loss of weight, we can use Aloe ferox as nutritional supplement for restoration of quantity and functions of basic tissues (*Dhatu*). All actions of this plant can help to improve absorption and assimilation of nutrients in all Seven Basic Tissues in the order and will also help for healing tissues of uterus and will improve the function of follicle-maturation. In some women, who have low growth in secondary sexual signs like breast development etc, this action can help to improve all over sexual development in these women.

Nutritional qualities of leaf pulp of Aloe ferox can help directly as supplement.

4. Balancing of humors –

As we have seen, leaf juice can be used as best regime for balancing the humors in our body. If we are using Bitters in treatment, then it should be used in discretion as it may cause *Pitta* and *Vata* aggravation in overdosage.

5. Antiparasitic and antimicrobial action –

Aloe ferox can show action as anti-parasitic (*Krumighna*) and as anti-microbial which can be used to treat conditions due to parasitic infestations or infections.

Aloe ferox as external treatment:

We can use Aloe ferox as ingredient in *Uttarbasti*.

Uttarbasti is the local *Ayurvedic* treatment in problems of female reproductive system which is used as a medicated enema administered in uterus.

Aloe ferox used in this, will help in many ways.

Aloe ferox can help as local cleanser for uterus and vagina by removing dead tissues, clots, secretions, excreta, toxins. It can be used as treatment for menstrual problems and also as postnatal care.

It can improve circulation of uterine endometrium and to improve contractions of uterus which allover works for inducing menses and for improving tone of uterus. It will help to remove aggravated humors and to alleviate remaining humors in uterus and other organs related to system. It can help to remove aggravated or vitiated *Pitta* causing inflammation and burning sensation, to remove aggravated or vitiated *Vata* humor which causes pain and aggravated or vitiated *Kapha* which causes heaviness and swelling according to *Ayurveda*. It can be also used as analgesic and anti-inflammatory herb.

It can also help as local treatment due to abnormal functions of uterus like lowered response of vessels, lowered tone of muscles which leads to abnormal menstrual bleeding patterns like less, heavy, normal bleeding with pain or menstruation with abnormal secretions like white discharge and pus. This can be used also as part of local treatment for abnormal growths in uterus.

Aloe bitters can be used as cleansers, emmenagogue and uterine stimulants while leaf juice can be used as local healing for vagina and uterus; as per condition requires.

Leaf juice can be used in enemas used for alleviation or soothing of the tissue inside.

Methods of treatment:
Aloe ferox can show various actions as mentioned above in treating menstrual problems like irregularities in period and flow, oligomenorrhea, amenorrhea, dysmenorrhea and infertility. Aloe ferox can be used as part of main treatment or maintenance treatment or prophylactic treatment.

Ayurveda recommends following types of treatments in *Yonivyapats.*

In conditions having severe bleeding, treatment comprises immediate control of bleeding and replenishing the blood and nutrients.

In conditions having chronic symptoms leading to chronic menstrual problems and infertility; thorough cleansing, balancing of humors and restoration of healthy menstruation with production of healthy ovum are the main steps in treatment.

If conditions are associated with pain, fever etc, then appropriate treatment is associated with herbs having actions against the specific symptom or group of symptoms.

We can use Cape Aloe or Aloe Bitters in very less dose like 100-300mg, depending upon general strength and severity of ailment, as oral administration or ingredient of *Uttarbasti.*

We can supplement Aloe ferox with some anti-inflammatory and analgesic herbs throughout this treatment.

We can use Cape Aloe or boiled and dried leaf juice of Aloe ferox in very less dose as part of internal or local treatment where cleansing, metabolism boost and improvement in general health is required. In conditions in menstrual problems due to general weakness, anemia and other debilitating diseases that require nourishment, leaf juice can be used in dosage from 10 ml to 30 ml as per strength of patient and severity of symptoms, as part of nourishment. We can use leaf juice of Aloe ferox.

In conditions that require local soothing or healing properties, leaf juice can be administered as part of *Uttarbasti* which will act as local anti-inflammatory, mild analgesic, tonic and anti-septic herb.

Aloe ferox can also help in irregular menses by correcting hormonal axis of body.

It can be used after delivery in very less dose as cleansing treatment or to ensure complete expulsion of placenta in patients having impaired uterine tone.

It can be used in secondary amenorrhea which means lack of menses after delivery for more than 3-4 months and even for longer period.

Caution:
Aloe ferox should be avoided in pregnant women as its use can cause abortions.

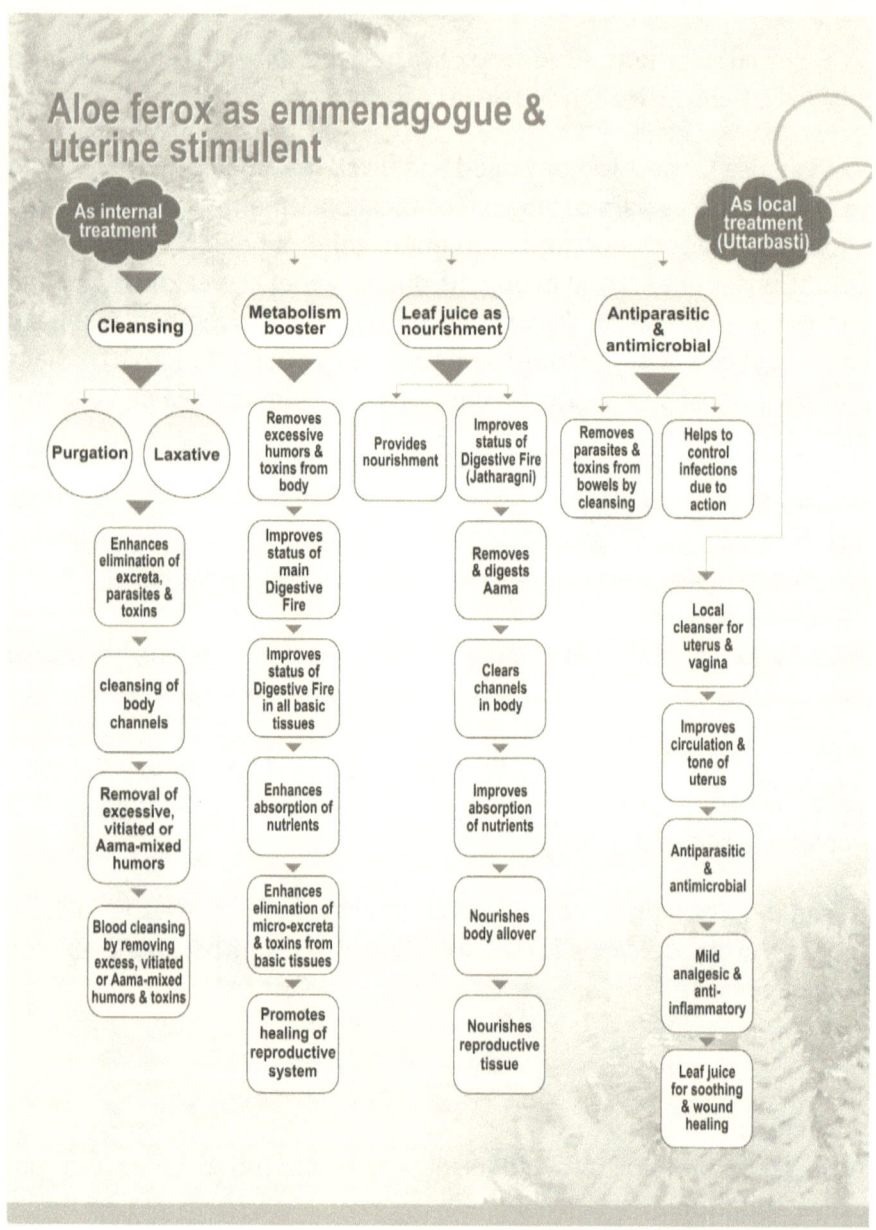

Aloe ferox as emmenagogue & uterine stimulent

As internal treatment

As local treatment (Uttarbasti)

Cleansing

Metabolism booster

Leaf juice as nourishment

Antiparasitic & antimicrobial

Purgation

Laxative

Removes excessive humors & toxins from body

Provides nourishment

Improves status of Digestive Fire (Jatharagni)

Removes parasites & toxins from bowels by cleansing

Helps to control infections due to action

Enhances elimination of excreta, parasites & toxins

Improves status of main Digestive Fire

Removes & digests Aama

Local cleanser for uterus & vagina

cleansing of body channels

Improves status of Digestive Fire in all basic tissues

Clears channels in body

Improves circulation & tone of uterus

Removal of excessive, vitiated or Aama-mixed humors

Enhances absorption of nutrients

Improves absorption of nutrients

Antiparasitic & antimicrobial

Blood cleansing by removing excess, vitiated or Aama-mixed humors & toxins

Enhances elimination of micro-excreta & toxins from basic tissues

Nourishes body allover

Mild analgesic & anti-inflammatory

Promotes healing of reproductive system

Nourishes reproductive tissue

Leaf juice for soothing & wound healing

Aloe ferox in skin diseases

Ayurvedic pathology of *Kustha* (Skin diseases)
Ayurvedic texts have given thorough information about anatomy and physiology of skin.

Skin diseases are collectively named as '*Kustha*'. There are main two types: *Mahakustha* (Leprosy) and *Kshudrakustha* (other skin diseases). Again these two types have subtypes on the basis of symptoms and have specific treatment. *Maha-kustha* has 7 subtypes while *Khsudra-kushtha* has 11 subtypes.

We will have look on pathology of skin diseases in short.

Skin diseases occur due to three main reasons: Improper diet habits, improper behavioral habits and Infections. Pathological process includes imbalance of humors, malnourishment of skin, accumulation of toxins in skin and adverse effects of those toxins in related tissues.

Pharmacological actions of Aloe ferox according to *Ayurveda*:

Aloe ferox as internal treatment:
Aloe ferox can be used as main treatment or as supplementary treatment as per requirement.

It can be a good combo-treatment for internal which serves broad spectrum of pharmacological actions and external treatment on various skin diseases as listed below:

1. Cleansing –
- **Purgation of accumulated excreta, parasites and toxins from body through bowels –** Due to purgative properties, Aloe Bitters can be used for thorough cleansing with proper care. This will help to remove all the excreta, toxins and parasites from bowels. This action can be helpful

in all types of skin diseases which need thorough internal cleansing of body through digestive system where it is applicable.

- **Cleansing of body channels along with micro-channels in skin** – Aloe ferox can help for cleansing the micro-channels in body. This action will help as general internal treatment in diseases which are caused by blockage of micro-channels (*Sookshma-srotas*) by micro-excreta (*Sookshma – mala* especially *Kleda* in relation to skin diseases), *Aama* or conditions occurred due to other factors like parasites or microorganisms. This also helps to establish normal flow of *Prana*, water, *RasaDhatu* and *RaktaDhatu* which helps to promote health of skin.

- **Removal of excessive and *Aama*-mixed or toxin-mixed humors** – If condition occurs due to aggravation or vitiation of humors, mild laxative properties of Aloe ferox can be used for a prolonged period. This action will also help for slow but constant removal of excessive, vitiated or *Aama*-mixed humors along with excreta and toxins produced due to imbalance in quantity and functions of humors.

- **Cleansing of blood** – We can use mild laxative action of Aloe ferox in skin diseases due to malfunction or vitiation of blood. This action will help for slow but constant removal of excessive, vitiated or *Aama*-mixed humors especially *Pitta* from blood which will ultimately help to remove root-cause.

- **Removes *Aama* from body** – It can help in all types of conditions occurring due to improper diet and activity routines which affect all the 13 types of 'Digestive Fire' explained in *Ayurvedic* texts, which cause production of *Aama* that obstructs all the channels in body and interferes with normal functions of humor. When *Aama* gets mixed with humors, it obstructs the nutrition of basic tissues which produces weak or abnormal tissues. In relation with skin diseases, this action will help to de-toxify the channels in layers of skin.

2. Metabolism booster –

Taste (*Rasa*), Post-digestive effect (*Vipak*) and Active energy (*Veerya*) along with its properties (*Gunas*) can help as effective medicine on associated symptoms like low appetite, digestion trouble, mal-absorption and ultimately malnutrition occurring due to altered functions of 13 types of 'Digestive Fire' in body. Though there are 13 types, other 12 types are dependent on main entity which is *Jatharagni* or 'Digestive Fire' situated in stomach, duodenum and pancreatic area.

Normal functions of this type of 'Digestive Fire' depend mainly on status of *Pitta* humor in body.

Aloe ferox helps to cleanse the micro and macro-channels in body, removes root cause of skin diseases which can be excessive and impure humors. This action can help to digest *Aama* and *Kleda* (by-product of metabolism of *Kapha* Humor which can cause obstruction if produced in excess). It can help to restore the functions of 'Digestive Fire' as well, which all over helps to improve the cellular level metabolism in skin.

3. Nourishment of *Dhatu* –

In conditions showing malnourishment and loss of weight, we can use Aloe ferox as nutritional supplement for restoration of quantity and functions of basic tissues (*Dhatu*). All actions of this plant can help to improve absorption and assimilation of nutrients in all basic tissues in the order and will also help for healing tissues of skin. Nourishment of *ShukraDhatu* and *Oja* also helps in maintenance o health of skin due to their relation to hormones as explained before.

Nutritional qualities of leaf pulp of Aloe ferox can help directly as supplement.

4. Balancing of humors –

As we have seen, leaf juice can be used as best regime for balancing the humors in our body. If we are using Bitters in treatment, then it should be used in discretion as it may cause *Pitta* and *Vata* aggravation in overdosage.

5. Antiparasitic and antimicrobial action –

Aloe ferox can show action as anti-parasitic (*Krumighna*) and as anti-microbial which can be used to treat conditions due to parasitic infestations or infections.

Aloe ferox as external treatment:

It can also be used as external treatment for various skin diseases as antiseptic and treating wounds.

It shows pharmacological actions to cleanse and heal skin lesions.

It provides a soothing, cool and anti-microbial application on various skin diseases with irritation and burning sensation.

We can use leaf juice of Aloe ferox internally and also for local treatment in skin diseases like Eczema, Scabies, Erysepalus, Leprosy and skin rashes due to various other infections.

It can be used in Diabetic sores and also in veneral sores.

Methods of treatment:

We can use bitters of Aloe for strong cleansing in severe cases of constipation and in strong patients to clean bowels with discretion.

For mild cleansing, bitters should be used in very low doses or leaf juice can be used.

For patients, who need follow-up treatment; can use leaf juice as supplement.

Leaf juice should be used for external application in form of swabs or Aloe bandages etc.

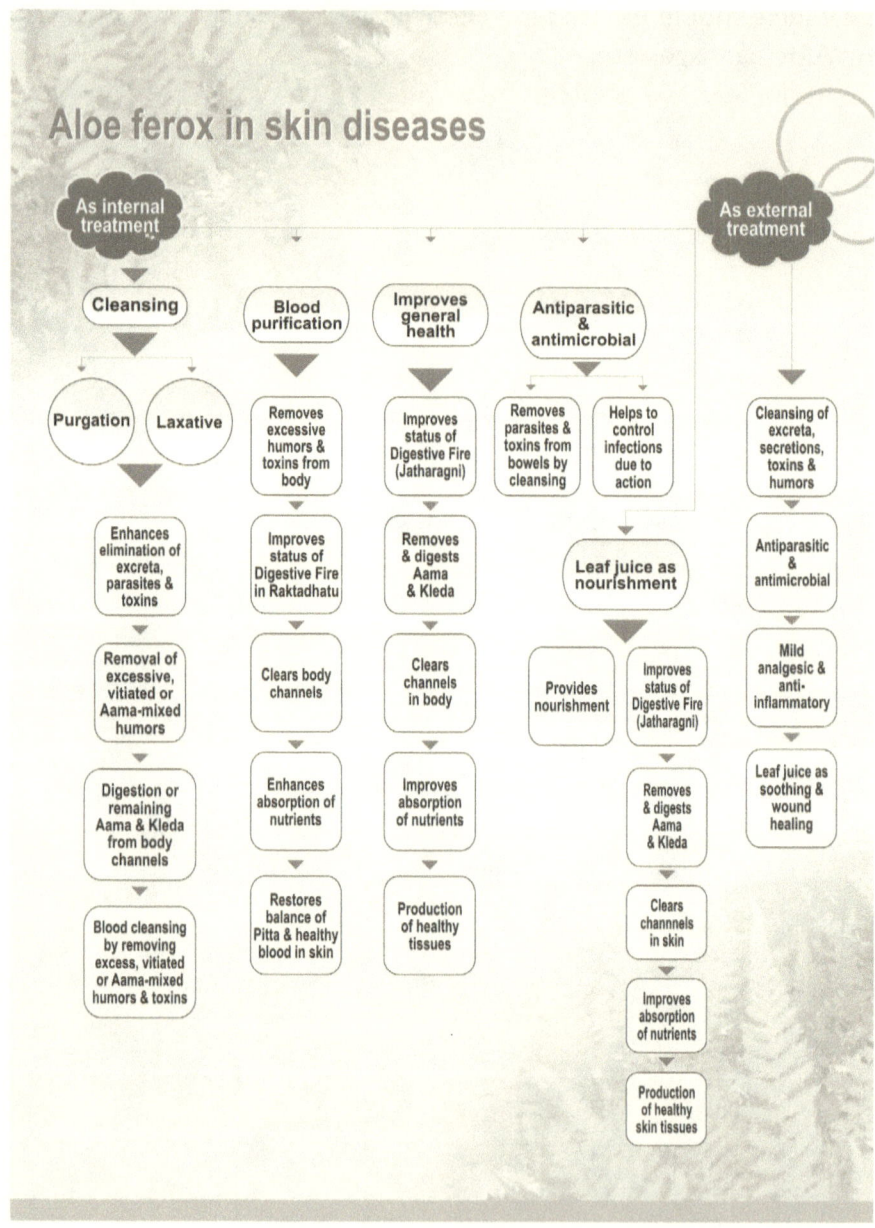

Aloe ferox in skin diseases

Aloe ferox for AIDS

Ayurvedic concept of AIDS:
Ayurvedic texts explain about a disease which has resembling etiological factors, symptoms and prognosis to AIDS. This disease is called as *'Pratilom Rajyakshma'*. This disease is mentioned as a type of *Rajyakshma* i.e. Tuberculosis. This throws light on the prevalence of Tuberculosis in HIV-infected and AIDS Patients in that time.

Main etiological factors are neglection of health, improper diet habits and irresponsible sexual behavior.

Symptoms are mainly those of Tuberculosis with severe tissue malnutrition. According to *Ayurvedic* Pathology, this disease show infection of reproductive tissue first and then affects other tissues gradually.

Pharmacological actions of Aloe ferox according to *Ayurveda*:
Aloe ferox can help as supportive treatment in HIV infected cases and AIDS Patients due to following actions:

Aloe ferox as internal treatment:
According to the qualities and pharmacological actions of Aloe ferox in *Ayurvedic* perspective, it can help in treatment of HIV and AIDS:

I. Cleansing –
- **Purgation of accumulated excreta, parasites and toxins from body through bowels –** Due to purgative properties, Aloe Bitters can be used for thorough cleansing with proper care. This will help to remove all the excreta, toxins and parasites from bowels.

- **Cleansing of body channels –** Aloe ferox can help for cleansing the micro-channels in body.

83

- **Removal of excessive and *Aama*-mixed or toxin-mixed humors** – If there is tendency to have abscesses due to aggravation or vitiation of humors, mild laxative properties of Aloe ferox can be used for a prolonged period. This action will also help for slow but constant removal of excessive, vitiated or *Aama*-mixed humors along with excreta and toxins produced due to imbalance in quantity and functions of humors. If there are symptoms due to vitiation of blood because of excessive, vitiated or *Aama*-mixed humors especially *Pitta*, then considering the relation of *Pitta* humor with blood, we can use Aloe ferox for mild laxative action which will help in related types of symptoms.

- **Cleansing of blood** – We can use mild laxative action of Aloe ferox in symptoms occurring due to malfunction or vitiation of blood. This action will help for slow but constant removal of excessive, vitiated or *Aama*-mixed humors especially *Pitta* from blood which will ultimately help to cure infections and will restore functions of internal organs.

- **Removes *Aama* from body** – It can help in all types of abscesses occurring due to improper diet and activity routines which affect all the 13 types of 'Digestive Fire' explained in *Ayurvedic* texts, which cause production of *Aama* that obstructs all the channels in body and interferes with normal functions of humor. When *Aama* gets mixed with humors, it causes wide range of symptoms, from bodyache-mild fever up to severe symptoms like failures of vital organs. This action of Aloe ferox as metabolism booster will help to remove *Aama* and *Aama*-mixed humors from micro-channels in body due to its qualities.

Cleansing action with all above aspects can be helpful for fast recovery from common infections.

2. Metabolism booster –
Taste (*Rasa*), Postdigestive effect (*Vipak*) and Active energy (*Veerya*) along with its properties (*Gunas*) can help as effective medicine

on associated symptoms like low appetite, digestion trouble, mal-absorption and ultimately malnutrition occurring due to altered functions of 13 types of 'Digestive Fire' in body. Though there are 13 types, other 12 types are dependent on main entity which is *Jatharagni* or 'Digestive Fire' situated in stomach, duodenum and pancreatic area.

Normal functions of this type of 'Digestive Fire' depend on status of *Pitta* humor in body.

Aloe ferox helps to cleanse the micro and macro-channels in body, removes root cause of all imbalances which can be excessive and impure humors. It can help to restore the functions of 'Digestive Fire' as well, which all over helps to improve the cellular level metabolism in body.

This will help ultimately as general health-booster and immunity-booster.

3. Nourishment of *Dhatu* –
In conditions showing malnourishment and loss of weight, we can use Aloe ferox as nutritional supplement for restoration of quantity and functions of basic tissues (*Dhatu*). All actions of this plant can help to improve absorption and assimilation of nutrients in all Seven Basic Tissues in the order which ultimately helps to nourish reproductive tissue (*ShukraDhatu*). This action can help in HIV infected and AIDS patients who show vitiation and depletion of *ShukraDhatu* predominantly according to *Ayurvedic* Pathology.

This action will also help for healing wounds and scars.

Nutritional qualities of leaf pulp of Aloe ferox can help directly as supplement.

4. Balancing of humors –
As we have seen, leaf juice can be used as best regime for balancing the humors in our body. If we are using Bitters in treatment, then it should be used in discretion as it may cause *Pitta* and *Vata* aggravation in overdosage.

5. Antiparasitic and antimicrobial action –

Aloe ferox can show action as anti-parasitic (*Krumighna*) and as anti-microbial which can be used to treat parasitic infestations or infections.

External treatment for wounds and sores –

It can also be used as external treatment for various external lesions as antiseptic and treating wounds.

Methods of treatment:

We can use Aloe bitters or Cape Aloe for thorough internal cleansing in HIV and AIDS patients which will help to avoid frequent infections and will also help in speedy recovery from common infections.

Leaf juice in small doses used internally as nutritional supplement in AIDS patients and HIV infected people can help to nourish all tissues and to increase immunity as well.

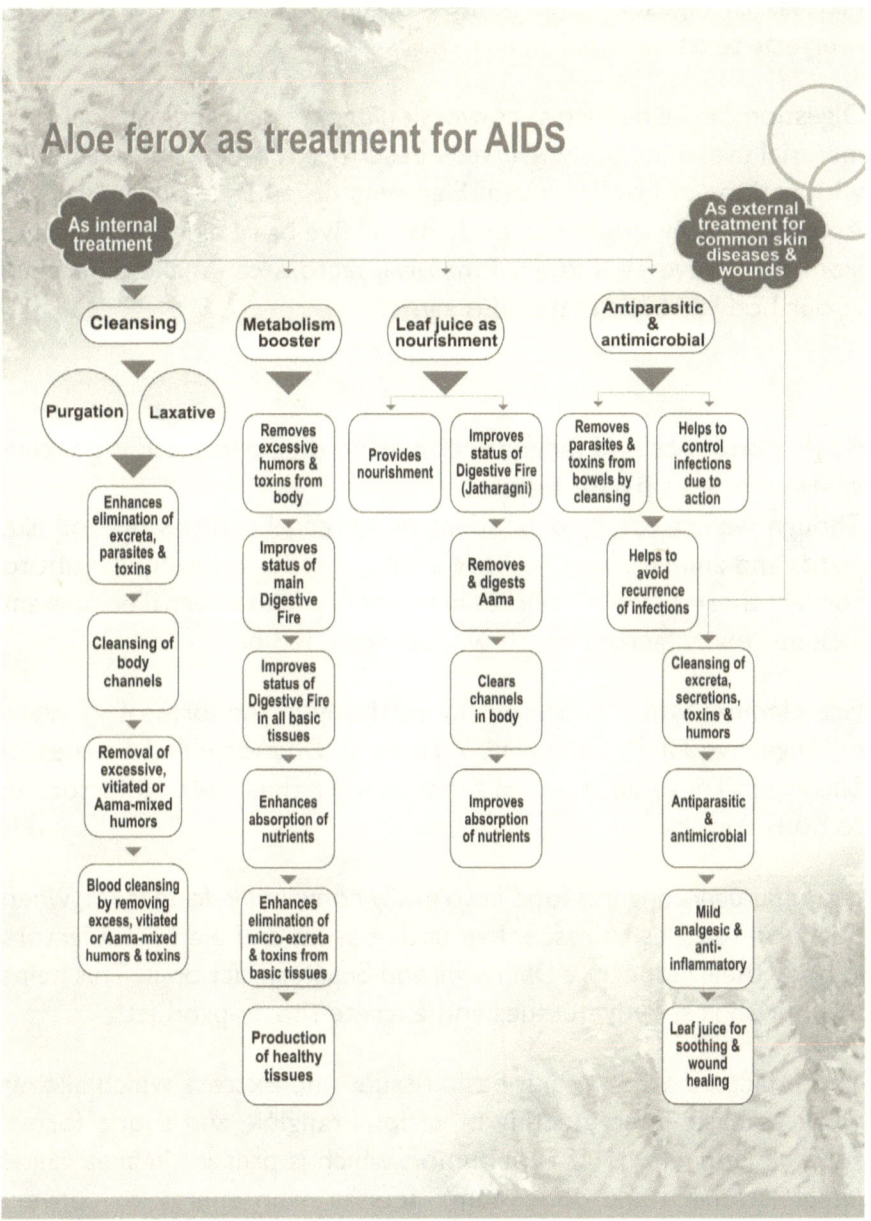

Aloe ferox as treatment for AIDS

As internal treatment

As external treatment for common skin diseases & wounds

Cleansing

Metabolism booster

Leaf juice as nourishment

Antiparasitic & antimicrobial

Purgation | **Laxative**

Enhances elimination of excreta, parasites & toxins

↓

Cleansing of body channels

↓

Removal of excessive, vitiated or Aama-mixed humors

↓

Blood cleansing by removing excess, vitiated or Aama-mixed humors & toxins

Removes excessive humors & toxins from body

↓

Improves status of main Digestive Fire

↓

Improves status of Digestive Fire in all basic tissues

↓

Enhances absorption of nutrients

↓

Enhances elimination of micro-excreta & toxins from basic tissues

↓

Production of healthy tissues

Provides nourishment

Improves status of Digestive Fire (Jatharagni)

↓

Removes & digests Aama

↓

Clears channels in body

↓

Improves absorption of nutrients

Removes parasites & toxins from bowels by cleansing

Helps to control infections due to action

↓

Helps to avoid recurrence of infections

↓

Cleansing of excreta, secretions, toxins & humors

↓

Antiparasitic & antimicrobial

↓

Mild analgesic & anti-inflammatory

↓

Leaf juice for soothing & wound healing

Aloe ferox for digestive troubles

Ayurvedic concept of digestive system and its function

Process of digestion and related organs are vividly described in *Ayurvedic* texts.

Digestion can be defined as conversion of external food material in to material useful for body. *Ayurveda* describes this concept beautifully with actions of Five Universal Elements called *Panchamahabhootas*. According to *Ayurveda*, our body has all five basic elemental factors from this Universe. External material factors can make difference in our body as basic material is same.

Basic concepts and factors related to digestion and digestive system are as listed below:

Though we are totally dependent on external sources of food like plants and animals, we also have a special capacity or equipment to convert these external sources in to energy. This internal equipment includes many factors which will be explained now.

Fire element which is present in our body in the form of 13 types of 'Digestive Fire' (*Jatharagni*, 7 types of *Dhatvagni* and 5 types of *Bhootagni*).These all types of fires convert their related factors in to body factors.

E.g. *Jatharagni* converts food in to easily convertible food form, when this food reaches to respective basic tissues and elemental factors in body their respective *Dhatvagni* and *Bhootagni* act on it. This helps to nourish respective tissues and excrete the by-products.

These factors are humors, basic tissues and excreta which allover work as basic energy acting in various tangible and subtle forms. *Paachak Pitta*, a type of *Pitta* humor, which is present in area called *Jathar* (stomach and duodenum), acts as main energy to convert solid food particles in to easily absorbable food form. *Kledak Kapha* in stomach helps to soften and moisten the food products and also protect lining of organs in *Jathar* from action of *Pitta* humor.

Three types of *Vata* humor help in process of digestion. *Samaan Vata* helps to control the action of 'Digestive Fire'. *Vyan Vata* distributes the nutrients allover our body while *Prana Vata* is the energy which helps our body to utilize these nutrients efficiently.

RasaDhatu and *RaktaDhatu* are the basic tissues which carry these nutrients from food to each and every cell with the help of *Vyan Vata* and allow cells to utilize those with the help of *Prana Vata*.

Basic organs related to function of digestion:
If we want to label the organs related to function of digestion in *Ayurvedic* aspect, then we will have encompass our whole body, mind and spirit.

Ayurveda describes rules of regulations about having proper diet which are collectively called as *'Ahaar-vidhi-visheshaayatana'*.

This guidance helps us to consider all five sense organs (tongue, nose, eyes, ears and skin) and our mind as well. Reactions of sense organs and mind are very important according to *Ayurveda*. Not only body organs but our soul is also important factor in acceptance of diet. *Ayurveda* provides us holistic guidance about choosing food which will be acceptable and beneficial for our body, mind and soul.

If we want to consider only body organs then *Ayurveda* explains all the organs from tongue till anus; anatomically and physiologically as well. Concepts called *Grahani* and *Annavahasrotas* are special concepts in *Ayurveda*. *Grahani* is mentioned as main site of 'Digestive Fire' which is anatomically located from stomach up to duodenum. Basic process of digestion starts and partially done in this are. *Ayurveda* says that *Grahani* is the site of *Pittadhara Kala* which is a special lining that performs function of digestion and absorption.

Annavahasrotas is a complex system including organs, macro and micro-channels in our body which distribute the nutrients on visible and subtle levels.

Major disorders of digestive system according to Ayurveda:

There are number of disorders explained in *Ayurvedic* texts due to imbalance of functions of digestive system. As *Ayurvedic* guidance explains about complex mechanism of nutrition in holistic view, we have to consider all the physical, mental and spiritual disorders due to violation of *Ayurvedic* rules of diet.

In that broad sense, all the symptoms of lack of nutrition, over nutrition and improper nutrition (nutrition in abnormal ways or abnormal factors) should be considered here.

Among this entire long list of symptoms and diseases, major ones are *Agnimandya* (weak 'Digestive Fire'), *Ajeerna* (indigestion), *AmlaPitta* (Symptoms due to increased acidity), *Parinaamshoola* (chronic pain due to imbalance in this system), *Atisaar* (diarrhea), *Chaardi* (vomiting), *Pravahika* (dyssentry), *Grahani* (chronic disorder showing lack of normal functions of digestion) are explained in detail with all possible etiological factors, pathological events, symptoms, prognosis and treatment.

Pharmacological actions of Aloe ferox according to Ayurveda:

According to the qualities and pharmacological actions of Aloe ferox in *Ayurvedic* perspective, we can use it as a tonic or function-enhancer for digestive system.

1. Cleansing –
  - **Purgation of accumulated excreta, parasites and toxins from body through bowels –** Due to purgative properties, Aloe Bitters can be used for thorough cleansing with proper care. This will help to remove all the excreta, toxins and parasites from bowels.

  - **Cleansing of body channels –** Aloe ferox can help for cleansing the micro-channels in body.

- **Removal of excessive and *Aama*-mixed or toxin-mixed humors –** If digestive disorders are due to aggravation or vitiation of humors especially due to *Aama*, mild laxative properties of Aloe ferox can be used for a prolonged period. This action will also help for slow but constant removal of excessive, vitiated or *Aama*-mixed humors along with excreta and toxins produced due to imbalance in quantity and functions of humors. If there are symptoms due to vitiation of blood because of excessive, vitiated or *Aama*-mixed humors especially *Pitta*, then considering the relation of *Pitta* humor with blood, we can use Aloe ferox for mild laxative action which will help in related types of symptoms.

- **Cleansing of blood –** We can use mild laxative action of Aloe ferox in symptoms occurring due to malfunction or vitiation of blood. This action will help for slow but constant removal of excessive, vitiated or *Aama*-mixed humors especially *Pitta* from blood which will ultimately help to cure infections and will restore functions of internal organs.

- **Removes *Aama* from body –** *Aama* is the main cause of many diseases in our body which should be removed as early as possible. Aloe ferox can help in symptoms and diseases occurring due to improper diet and activity routines which affect all the 13 types of 'Digestive Fire' explained in *Ayurvedic* texts, which cause production of *Aama* that obstructs all the channels in body and interferes with normal functions of humor. When *Aama* gets mixed with humors, it causes wide range of symptoms, from bodyache-mild fever up to severe symptoms like failures of vital organs. This action of Aloe ferox as metabolism booster will help to remove *Aama* and *Aama*-mixed humors from micro-channels in body due to its qualities.

Cleansing action with all above aspects can be helpful for fast recovery from common infections of system.

2. Metabolism booster –
Taste (*Rasa*), Postdigestive effect (*Vipak*) and Active energy (*Veerya*) along with its properties (*Gunas*) can help as effective medicine on symptoms like low appetite, digestion trouble, mal-absorption and ultimately malnutrition occurring due to altered functions of 13 types of 'Digestive Fire' in body. Though there are 13 types, other 12 types are dependent on main entity which is *Jatharagni* or 'Digestive Fire' situated in stomach, duodenum and pancreatic area.

Normal functions of this type of 'Digestive Fire' depend on status of *Pitta* humor in body.

Aloe ferox helps to cleanse the micro and macro-channels in body, removes root cause of all imbalances which can be excessive and impure humors. It can be good activator for organs like liver, gall bladder and intestines to secret more digestive juices.

It can help to restore the functions of 'Digestive Fire' as well, which allover help to improve appetite, digestion and assimilation of nutrients. This can also help as General health booster and immunity booster by improving the cellular level metabolism in body.

3. Nourishment of *Dhatu* –
In conditions showing malnourishment and loss of weight, we can use Aloe ferox as nutritional supplement for restoration of quantity and functions of basic tissues (*Dhatu*). All actions of this plant can help to improve absorption and assimilation of nutrients in all Seven Basic Tissues in the order and will also help for healing our body inside out.

Nutritional qualities of leaf pulp of Aloe ferox can help directly as supplement.

4. Balancing of humors –
As we have seen, leaf juice can be used as best regime for balancing the humors in our body where it is necessary. If we are using Bitters in treatment, then it should be used in discretion as it may cause *Pitta* and *Vata* aggravation in overdosage.

5. Antiparasitic and antimicrobial action –

Aloe ferox can show action as anti-parasitic (*Krumighna*) and as anti-microbial which can be used to treat intestinal parasitic infestations or infections.

Methods of treatment:

Aloe ferox can be used as main treatment in symptoms or diseases of digestive system or as assisting treatment to main treatment. It can be used as prophylactic treatment for avoiding any digestive trouble in advance or also as after-treatment to the main treatment for digestive disorders.

It can be used as supplement for some major chronic illnesses like tuberculosis, diabetes, AIDS etc.

We can use Aloe bitters or Cape Aloe as cleanser in low doses for a certain period as per strength of patients and severity of symptoms.

As a next step, leaf pulp can be used as nourishment.

It can be a good bitter tonic in all major chronic illnesses.

In HIV infected and AIDS patients who show vitiation and depletion of *ShukraDhatu* predominantly according to *Ayurvedic* Pathology.

We can use leaf sap of Aloe ferox as tonic in very low doses to improve quality of digestion and absorption in people having chronic digestive disturbances due to improper and irregular diet, addictions, improper functions of liver and also due to chronic constipation.

It can be a help for people having diabetes and also for people having low appetite and digestion due to chronic medications.

Caution:

Aloe ferox should be avoided in pregnant women as its use can cause abortions.

93

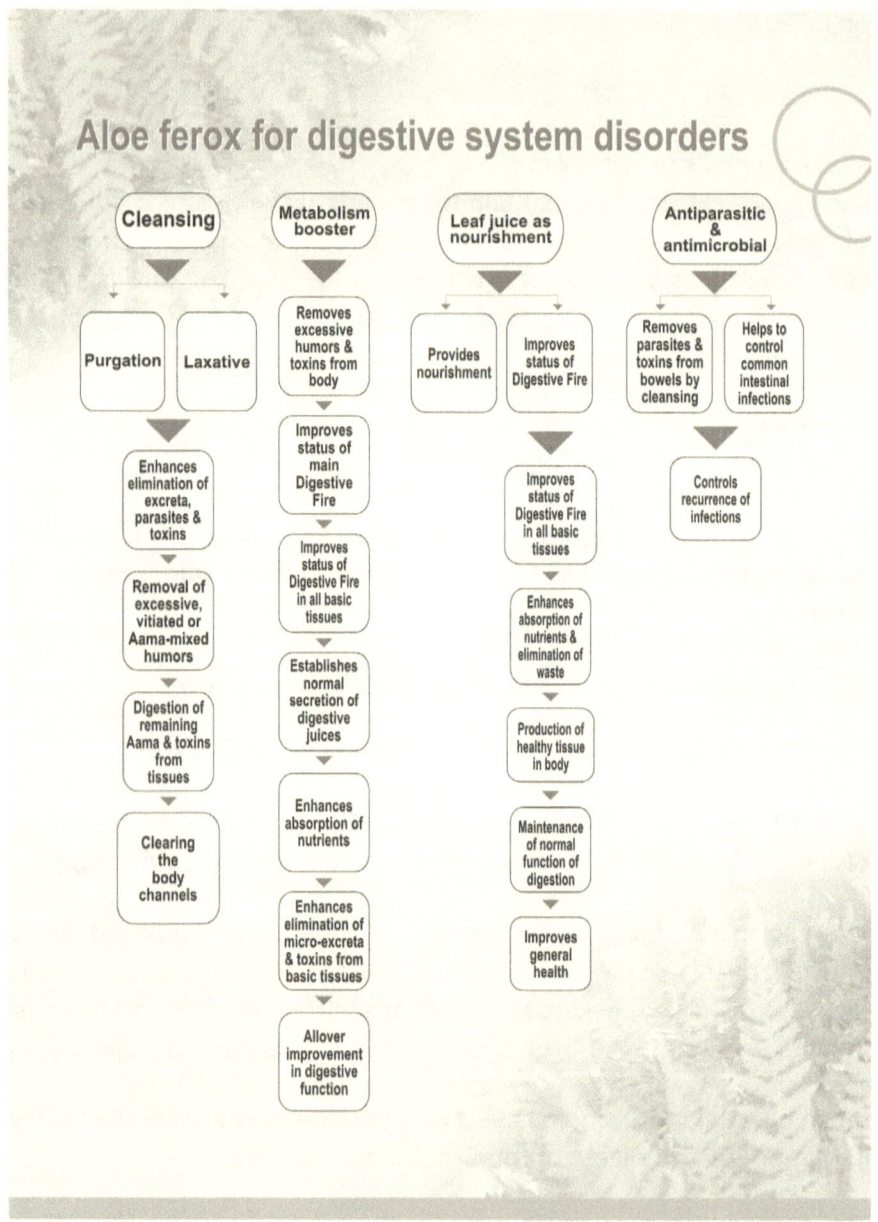

Aloe ferox for digestive system disorders

Aloe ferox for gout

Ayurvedic concept of 'Gout'

Ayurvedic texts explain in detail about a disease which has close resemblance to gout and that disease is '*Vatarakta*'. This word '*Vatarakta*' is made of two words; *Vata* means *Vata* humor and *Rakta* means blood. According to *Ayurveda*, this disease occurs due to vitiation of *Vata* humor and blood due to their own etiological factors and together these two factors cause *Vatarakta*.

Etiological factors point towards improper diet and activities which manly aggravate *Vata* humor and vitiate blood.

Symptoms are similar to those of gout though pathological process is explained in different way.

Line of treatment emphasizes mainly on thorough cleansing and alleviation of humors to control swelling and pain in joints.

Ayurvedic types of gout

Ayurvedic texts explain about 4 major types of this disease based on predominance of humors:

Vatadhik – Predominantly *Vata* humor vitiation

Pittadhik – Predominantly *Pitta* humor vitiation

Kaphadhik – Predominantly *Kapha* humor vitiation

Raktadhik – Predominantly blood vitiation

Two stages of this disease are mentioned:

Uttan – Superficial tissues like skin and muscles get affected.

Gambhir – Deep tissues like bones, joints and marrow are affected.

Pharmacological actions of Aloe ferox according to *Ayurveda*:

Aloe ferox can be used as part of internal treatment or external application for *Vatarakta* or gout.

Internal treatment:

According to the qualities and pharmacological actions of Aloe ferox in *Ayurvedic* perspective, we can use it as main treatment or supplementary treatment for gout.

I. Cleansing –

- **Purgation of accumulated excreta, parasites and toxins from body through bowels** – Due to purgative properties, Aloe Bitters can be used for thorough cleansing with proper care. This will help to remove all the excreta, toxins and parasites from bowels.

- **Cleansing of body channels** – Aloe ferox can help for cleansing the micro-channels in body.

- **Removal of excessive and *Aama*-mixed or toxin-mixed humors** – If digestive disorders are due to aggravation or vitiation of humors especially due to *Aama*, mild laxative properties of Aloe ferox can be used for a prolonged period. This action will also help for slow but constant removal of excessive, vitiated or *Aama*-mixed humors along with excreta and toxins produced due to imbalance in quantity and functions of humors. If there are symptoms due to vitiation of blood because of excessive, vitiated or *Aama*-mixed humors especially *Pitta*, then considering the relation of *Pitta* humor with blood, we can use Aloe ferox for mild laxative action which will help in related types of symptoms.

- **Cleansing of blood –** As pathological process of *Vatarakta* or gout includes vitiation of blood, blood cleansing action of Aloe ferox can be a major part of treatment. We can use mild laxative action of Aloe ferox in symptoms occurring due to malfunction or vitiation of blood. This action will help for slow but constant removal of excessive, vitiated or *Aama*-mixed humors especially *Pitta* from blood which will ultimately help to cure infections and will restore functions of internal organs.

- **Removes *Aama* from body –** *Aama* is one of the major factors in pathological processes of joint problems, which should be removed as early as possible. Aloe ferox can help in *Vatarakta* where *Aama* is also present due to improper diet and activity routines. This action of Aloe ferox as metabolism booster will help to remove *Aama* and *Aama*-mixed humors from micro-channels in body due to its qualities.

Cleansing action with all above aspects can be helpful for fast recovery.

2. Metabolism booster –

Taste (*Rasa*), Postdigestive effect (*Vipak*) and Active energy (*Veerya*) along with its properties (*Gunas*) can help as effective medicine on symptoms like low appetite, digestion trouble, mal-absorption and ultimately malnutrition occurring due to altered functions of 13 types of 'Digestive Fire' in body. Though there are 13 types, other 12 types are dependent on main entity which is *Jatharagni* or 'Digestive Fire' situated in stomach, duodenum and pancreatic area.

Normal functions of this type of 'Digestive Fire' depend on status of *Pitta* humor in body.

Aloe ferox helps to cleanse the micro and macro-channels in body, removes root cause of all imbalances which can be excessive and impure humors. It can be good activator for organs like liver, gall bladder and intestines to secret more digestive juices.

It can help to restore the functions of 'Digestive Fire' as well, which allover help to improve appetite, digestion and assimilation of nutrients. This can also help as general health booster and immunity booster by improving the cellular level metabolism in body.

3. Maintaining of balance of humors –

Cleansing action removes excessive and vitiated humors while qualities like *Rasa, Veerya, Vipak* as explained in chapter No. 4 help in balancing the humors if required further.

Removal of vitiated and excessive *Vata* along with *Vata* alleviating qualities of Aloe ferox will help to reduce *Vata* - related symptoms like sharp pain, joint stiffness etc.

Removal of vitiated and excessive *Pitta* along with *Pitta* alleviating qualities of Aloe ferox will help to reduce *Pitta* - related symptoms like inflammation, burning sensation etc.

Removal of vitiated and excessive *Kapha* along with *Kapha* alleviating qualities of Aloe ferox will help to reduce *Kapha* - related symptoms like swelling, heaviness etc.

4. Nourishment of *Dhatu* –

In conditions showing malnourishment and loss of weight, we can use Aloe ferox as nutritional supplement for restoration of quantity and functions of basic tissues (*Dhatu*). All actions of this plant can help to improve absorption and assimilation of nutrients in all Seven Basic Tissues in the order and will also help for healing our body inside out.

Nutritional qualities of leaf pulp of Aloe ferox can help directly as supplement.

5. Antiparasitic and antimicrobial action –

Aloe ferox can show action as anti-parasitic (*krumighna*) and as anti-microbial which can be used for treatment of intestinal parasitic infestations or infections.

External treatment –
It can also be used as external treatment in form of packs or poultices. It can provide a soothing, cool and anti-microbial application which will be a good local treatment for swollen and painful joints in gout.

Methods of treatment:
Aloe ferox can be used as part of main treatment or maintenance treatment or prophylactic treatment.

We need to supplement Aloe ferox with some herbs having predominantly anti-inflammatory and analgesic action throughout this treatment in severely inflamed joints.

We can use Aloe ferox in packs or poultices as a drawing agent which will draw local toxins and vitiated humors in the area of inflammation and then *Raktamokshan* (blood letting) with proper care.

We can use leaf juice of Aloe ferox as dressing on the wound as well.

We can use Cape Aloe or boiled and dried leaf juice of Aloe ferox in very less dose for first step i.e. internal cleansing.

Use of Aloe ferox internally in low doses can help as good prophylactic treatment for gout.

In addition to proper treatment, *Ayurveda* recommends avoiding too much protein food, alcohol, salty-pungent and food having hot property e.g. spices, daytime sleep, too much exercise, working near fire or in too hot areas e.g. working near furnaces.

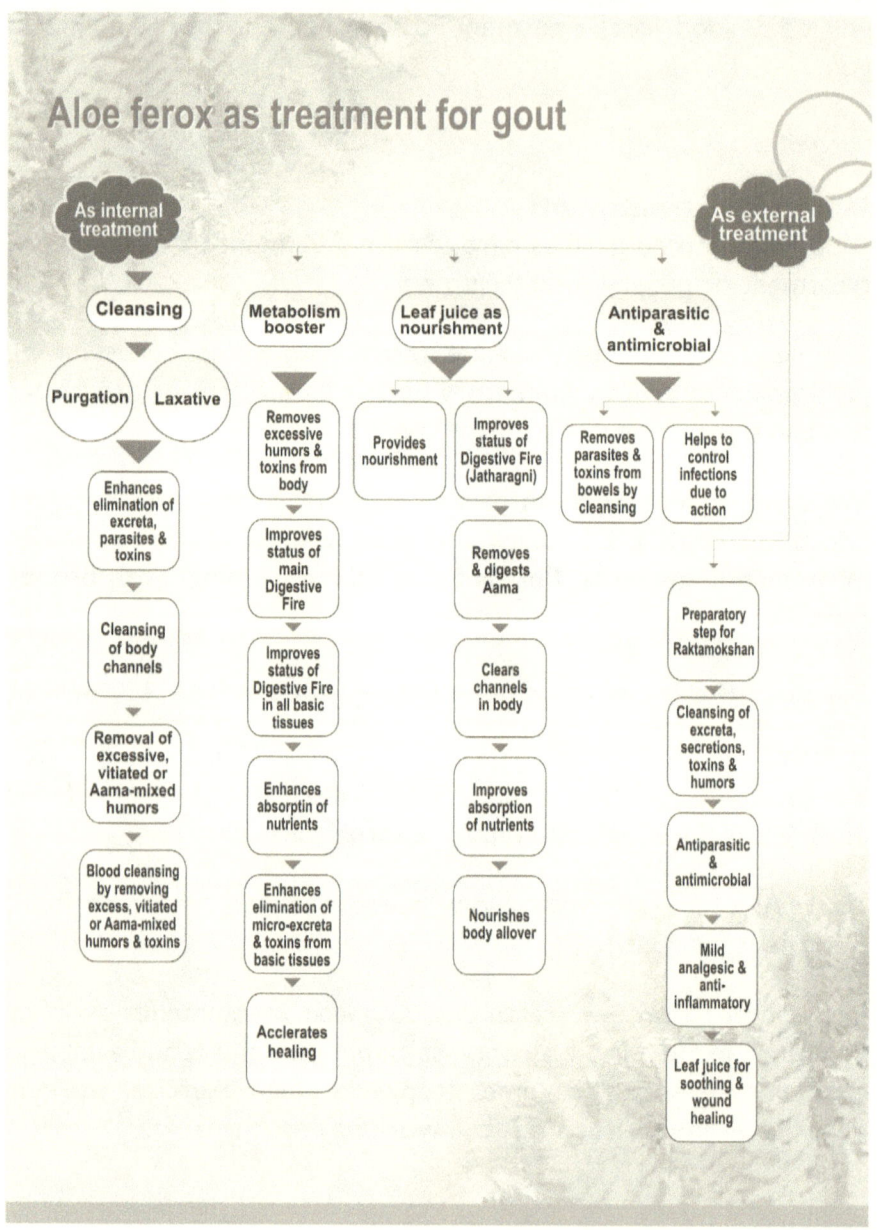

Aloe ferox as treatment for gout

Aloe ferox for anemia

Ayurvedic explanation of anemia:
Ayurveda names this disease as 'Pandu' which is a noun in the ancient Indian language, Sanskrit having meaning 'white' or 'pale'.

Skin of anemic patients looks pale and lusterless which is the most visible sign when we first see these cases. Ayurvedic Gurus have explained synonyms of this disease, types of this disease, etiological factors, pathological process, symptoms, signs, prognosis and treatment of all the various types.

Main etiological factors are as follows:
Improper diet, improper activity routine (especially too much exertion) which causes imbalance in body, factors affecting psychological health and a specific factor mentioned is 'Pica or habit of eating soil'.

Systems affected in this pathology are Rasavahasrotas and Raktavahasrotas which work together to provide nourishment to allover body.

Line of treatment is decided on the basis of etiological factor, pathological process and severity of symptoms.

In general, treatment of anemia includes following steps:

- Cleansing of body
- Restoration of 'Digestive Fire'
- Balancing basic humors
- Anti-parasitic and anti-microbial treatments
- Surgical methods to correct etiological factors like trauma, wounds, haemorrhoids etc
- Replenishing basic tissues mainly RasaDhatu and RaktaDhatu by using various methods
- Nourishing all basic tissues to restore general strength and immunity as prophylactic measure.

Pharmacological actions of Aloe ferox according to Ayurveda:

We can use Aloe ferox as part of cleansing treatment or as a supportive treatment for main treatment.

We can use exudate (*Niryas*), solid extract of leaves (*Saar*) and leaf juice (*Patra-swaras*) of Aloe ferox for various types of anemia with discretion.

It can help in following ways:

I. Cleansing –

*   **Purgation of accumulated excreta, parasites and toxins from body through bowels –** Due to purgative properties, Aloe Bitters can be used for thorough cleansing with proper care. This will help to remove all the excreta, toxins and parasites from bowels.

*   **Cleansing of body channels –** Aloe ferox can help for cleansing the micro-channels in body as obstruction in channels is also one of the etiological factors.

*   **Removal of excessive and *Aama*-mixed or toxin-mixed humors –** If digestive disorders are due to aggravation or vitiation of humors especially due to *Aama*, mild laxative properties of Aloe ferox can be used for a prolonged period. This action will also help for slow but constant removal of excessive, vitiated or *Aama*-mixed humors along with excreta and toxins produced due to imbalance in quantity and functions of humors. Especially when blood gets vitiated because of excessive, vitiated or *Aama*-mixed humors especially *Pitta*, then considering the relation of *Pitta* humor with blood, we can use Aloe ferox for mild laxative action which will help in related types of symptoms.

*   **Cleansing of blood –** We can use mild laxative action of Aloe ferox in symptoms occurring due to malfunction or vitiation of blood. This action will help for slow but

constant removal of excessive, vitiated or *Aama*-mixed humors especially *Pitta* from blood which will ultimately help to cure infections and will restore functions of organs related to production of healthy blood tissue.

- **Removes *Aama* from body** – Aloe ferox can help in consitions where *Aama* is also present due to improper diet and activity routines. This action of Aloe ferox as metabolism booster will help to remove *Aama* and *Aama*-mixed humors from micro-channels in body due to its qualities.

Cleansing action with all above aspects can be helpful for fast recovery.

2. Metabolism booster –

Taste (*Rasa*), Postdigestive effect (*Vipak*) and Active energy (*Veerya*) along with its properties (*Gunas*) can help as effective medicine on symptoms like low appetite, digestion trouble, mal-absorption and ultimately malnutrition occurring due to altered functions of 13 types of 'Digestive Fire' in body. Though there are 13 types, other 12 types are dependent on main entity which is *Jatharagni* or 'Digestive Fire' situated in stomach, duodenum and pancreatic area.

Normal functions of this type of 'Digestive Fire' depend on status of *Pitta* humor in body.

Aloe ferox helps to cleanse the micro and macro-channels in body, removes root cause of all imbalances which can be excessive and impure humors. It can be good activator for organs like liver, gall bladder and intestines to secret more digestive juices.

It can help to restore the functions of 'Digestive Fire' as well, which allover help to improve appetite, digestion and assimilation of nutrients. This can also help as general health booster and immunity booster by improving the cellular level metabolism in body.

3. As a tonic for organs involved in pathological process of anemia –

Aloe ferox can work as anti-inflammatory (*Shothaghna*) and excellent tonic for improving functions of organs like liver, spleen, pancreas, intestines etc which are said to be directly and indirectly involved in action of 'Digestive Fire'.

It will remove obstruction in channels (*Srotorodha*) especially in type of anemia caused by Pica (habit of eating soil or any type of earthern matter).

It can also work as booster for metabolism of those systems which will help for better absorption of Iron and other nutrients which are essential for maintaining normal blood production in our body. .

This can be used as supplement for treatment of all types of anemia and also as prophylactic treatment.

It can be used as supplementary treatment in anemia for improving function of liver which is mentioned as one of the main sites of action for *Raktavahasrotas* and also as booster for action of *RaktaDhatvagni* ('Digestive Fire' in blood).

4. Balancing of humors –

As we have seen, leaf juice can be used as best regime for balancing the humors in our body. If we are using Bitters in treatment, then it should be used in discretion as it may cause *Pitta* and *Vata* aggravation in overdosage.

5. Nourishment of *Dhatu* –

In conditions showing malnourishment and loss of weight, we can use Aloe ferox as nutritional supplement for restoration of quantity and functions of basic tissues (*Dhatu*). All actions of this plant can help to improve absorption and assimilation of nutrients in all *Dhatus* in the order and will also help for healing our body inside out.

Nutritional qualities of leaf pulp of Aloe ferox can help directly as supplement.

6. Antiparasitic and antimicrobial action –

Aloe ferox can show action as anti-parasitic (*krumighna*) and as anti-microbial which can be used to treat intestinal parasitic infestations or infections.

Methods of treatment:

We can use Aloe Bitters or Cape Aloe for cleansing with proper inunction (Snehan) and care. It can be used frequently with breaks till we get signs of improved functions of Raktavaha srotas and general health.

In weak patients, dosage can be reduced as required or leaf juice can be given as mild laxative and general cleanser.

We can use leaf juice of Aloe ferox as supplementary treatment in patients taking complete treatment for anemia.

Leaf juice can be used in children as antiparasitic, general cleanser, metabolism booster and nutritional supplement with proper care and only under expert guidance.

Caution:

Aloe ferox should not be used in pregnant women as it can cause abortions.

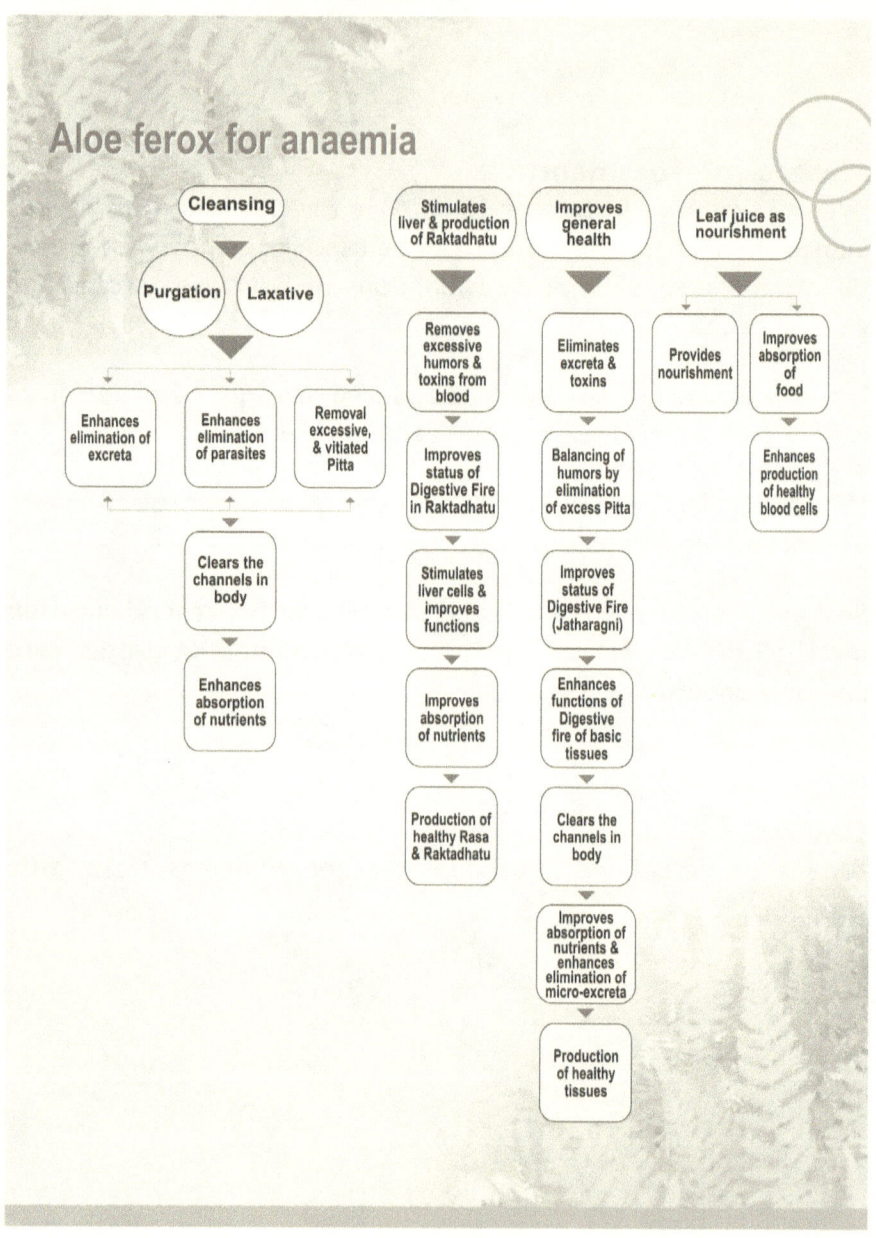

Aloe ferox for anaemia

Cleansing

Purgation | **Laxative**

Enhances elimination of excreta

Enhances elimination of parasites

Removal excessive, & vitiated Pitta

Clears the channels in body

Enhances absorption of nutrients

Stimulates liver & production of Raktadhatu

Removes excessive humors & toxins from blood

Improves status of Digestive Fire in Raktadhatu

Stimulates liver cells & improves functions

Improves absorption of nutrients

Production of healthy Rasa & Raktadhatu

Improves general health

Eliminates excreta & toxins

Balancing of humors by elimination of excess Pitta

Improves status of Digestive Fire (Jatharagni)

Enhances functions of Digestive fire of basic tissues

Clears the channels in body

Improves absorption of nutrients & enhances elimination of micro-excreta

Production of healthy tissues

Leaf juice as nourishment

Provides nourishment

Improves absorption of food

Enhances production of healthy blood cells

Aloe ferox for spleen problems

Ayurvedic description about spleen
Ayurveda has mentioned about spleen along with liver as they are close in abdominal cavity and *Ayurvedic* term for this organ is *'Pleeha'*. It is mentioned to be an important organ and has mentioned about anatomy and physiology of spleen with interesting details.

One of the important *Marmas* (Vital point) –
It is also counted in one of the very important *Marmas* which can cause death as name *'Pranahar Marma'* suggests (vital points in body). Name of that *Marma* is *'BruhatiSiraMarma'*. If a person gets hurt here, it leads to death after some time as this leads to severe bleeding through *'Sira-Marma'* or major vessels located here.

Importance of spleen in maintenance of production and functions of blood is mentioned along with liver everywhere in *Ayurvedic* texts.

Formation of spleen according to *Ayurvedic* Embryology –
As explained before, *Ayurvedic* Embryology (*Garbhaavakranti*) shows amazing explanation about every step in growth of intrauterine life and like liver, spleen is also produced by subtle changes occurring in metabolism of blood after fertilization. Though form of spleen can be seen later as well in intrauterine life, its relation to blood is also established at the exact time when embryo is in the form of tiny ball of cells like liver. Anatomical position of spleen is mentioned as close position below the heart.

Main organ in system producing and circulating blood –
Like liver, spleen also has importance as one of the main sites of action related to *Raktavahasrotas* or system which is involved in production and circulation of blood. Spleen is the site where *RasaDhatu* gets converted in to *RaktaDhatu* i.e. blood.

Relation of spleen to *Pitta* humor –
Spleen is the site where blood gets its red colour which according to *Ayurveda* is called *'Ranjan Karma'*. Blood is main site for action of *Ranjak Pitta*, a type of *Pitta* related to production of blood and that

is why, spleen is also related to *Pitta* humor due to its position as main site for this function of blood production.

That is why, if there is any disturbance or imbalance in metabolism of *Pitta* humor, it also affects spleen via blood and vice versa.

Pitta humor is the main energy behind the food metabolism in body. If there is any imbalance in this humor, it causes malfunctioning of blood and ultimately in related organs like liver and spleen. In the same way, if there is any imbalance or vitiation of blood or any spleen problem, then it affects food metabolism of body.

Main site for *Raktadharakala* –
As mentioned before, *Acharya Sushruta* has mentioned about a very special concept called '*Kala*' which is a membrane or group of tissues covering the cavities in related organs to perform very special and subtle functions in metabolism of all factors forming body.

Spleen has *Raktadharakala* (Membrane or tissues covering the cavities in related organs which deal with production and function of blood). That is why, according to *Ayurveda*, spleen plays important role in absorption and assimilation of nutrients, production of blood, maintaining healthy quantity and functions of blood and last but important function is, separation of nutrients from excreta while maintaining quantity of body nutrients in blood at healthy level.

Etiological factors and symptoms of spleen disorders according to *Ayurveda*
As *Ayurveda* considers spleen as part of a delicate balance of humors, basic tissues and micro-metabolisms, any imbalance in spleen affects nutrition and blood production.

If a person constantly continues having bad diet habits like eating food which is too much spicy or heat producing (vidahi), toxic, too much secretion-producing food (*Abhishyandi*), stale food, too much of indulgence in excessive alcohol etc and also continues with irresponsible, reckless lifestyle, addictions, then this aggravates or vitiates *Pitta*. Some infections especially acute or chronic fevers like typhoid, malaria mentioned as *Vishamjvar, Jeernajvar* in *Ayurveda* or physical trauma can also cause spleen problems.

Maharshi Charak has explained 5 types of spleen diseases on the basis of etiological factors;

Vata-predominance *(Vataj)*, *Pitta*-predominance *(Pittaj)*, *Kapha*-predominance *(Kaphaj)*, all three humors –predominance *(Sannipatik)* and Blood vitiation- predominance *(Raktaj)*

Symptoms of all these diseases show typical aggravation or vitiation symptoms of related humor *(Dosha)* or basic tissue *(Dhatu)*. But all of these conditions show splenomegaly and pain. If neglected they can lead to anemia, jaundice, ascitis, hemorrhage and abscess or growths. In types of ascitis, there is type in which spleen disorder is main cause and that type is named as *'Pleehodar'*.

One should treat these symptoms carefully after considering relation of spleen to humors *(Dosha)* and basic tissues *(Dhatu)* especially blood.

In conditions like aggravation or vitiation of *Pitta* humor by other excessive humors, toxins produced by microorganisms or *Aama* and symptoms of altered quality and quantity of blood (excluding internal or external blood loss), a proper checkup for assessment of function of spleen should be done and treated along with as part of main treatment and prophylactic treatment.

Considering relation of *Pitta*, blood and spleen according to *Ayurveda*, patients showing symptoms of altered functions of *Raktavahasrotas* also show symptoms of spleen disorder and should be treated with discretion and in line with general spleen disorders.

Pharmacological actions of Aloe ferox according to Ayurveda:
We can use Aloe ferox as part of cleansing treatment or as a supportive treatment for main treatment.

We can use exudate (*Niryas*), solid extract of leaves (*Saar*) and leaf juice (*Patraswaras*) of Aloe ferox for various types of anemia with discretion.

It can help in following ways:

I. Cleansing –
- **Purgation of accumulated excreta, parasites and toxins from body through bowels –** Due to purgative properties, Aloe Bitters can be used for thorough cleansing with proper care. This will help to remove all the excreta, toxins and parasites from bowels.

- **Cleansing of body channels –** Aloe ferox can help for cleansing the micro-channels in body as obstruction in channels is also one of the etiological factors.

- **Removal of excessive and *Aama*-mixed or toxin-mixed humors –** If digestive disorders are due to aggravation or vitiation of humors especially due to *Aama*, mild laxative properties of Aloe ferox can be used for a prolonged period. This action will also help for slow but constant removal of excessive, vitiated or *Aama*-mixed humors along with excreta and toxins produced due to imbalance in quantity and functions of humors. Especially when blood gets vitiated because of excessive, vitiated or *Aama*-mixed humors especially *Pitta*, then considering the relation of *Pitta* humor with blood, we can use Aloe ferox for mild laxative action which will help in related types of symptoms.

- **Cleansing of blood –** We can use mild laxative action of Aloe ferox in symptoms occurring due to malfunction or vitiation of blood. This action will help for slow but constant removal of excessive, vitiated or *Aama*-mixed humors especially *Pitta* from blood which will ultimately help to cure infections and will restore functions of organs related to production of healthy blood tissue.

- **Removes *Aama* from body** – Aloe ferox can help in conditions where *Aama* is also present due to improper diet and activity routines. This action of Aloe ferox as metabolism booster will help to remove *Aama* and *Aama*-mixed humors from micro-channels in body due to its qualities.

Cleansing action with all above aspects can be helpful for fast recovery.

2. Metabolism booster –

Taste (*Rasa*), Postdigestive effect (*Vipak*) and Active energy (*Veerya*) along with its properties (*Gunas*) can help as effective medicine on symptoms like low appetite, digestion trouble, mal-absorption and ultimately malnutrition occurring due to altered functions of 13 types of 'Digestive Fire' in body. Though there are 13 types, other 12 types are dependent on main entity which is *Jatharagni* or 'Digestive Fire' situated in stomach, duodenum and pancreatic area.

Normal functions of this type of 'Digestive Fire' depend on status of *Pitta* humor in body.

Aloe ferox helps to cleanse the micro and macro-channels in body, removes root cause of all imbalances which can be excessive and impure humors. It can be good activator for organs like liver, gall bladder and intestines to secret more digestive juices.

It can help to restore the functions of 'Digestive Fire' as well, which allover help to improve appetite, digestion and assimilation of nutrients. This can also help as general health booster and immunity booster by improving the cellular level metabolism in body.

3. Balancing of humors –

As we have seen, leaf juice can be used as best regime for balancing the humors in our body. This can be helpful in managing spleen disorders caused due to imbalance of humors. If we are using Bitters in treatment, then it should be used in discretion as it may cause *Pitta* and *Vata* aggravation in overdosage.

4. Nourishment of *Dhatu* –
In conditions showing malnourishment and loss of weight, we can use Aloe ferox as nutritional supplement for restoration of quantity and functions of basic tissues (*Dhatu*). All actions of this plant can help to improve absorption and assimilation of nutrients in all basic tissues in the order and will also help for healing our body inside out. This can also help in healing spleen tissue and work as a tonic for that specific organ due to its action on blood.

Nutritional qualities of leaf pulp of Aloe ferox can help directly as supplement.

5. Antiparasitic and antimicrobial action –
Aloe ferox can show action as anti-parasitic (*krumighna*) and as anti-microbial which can be used for the treatment of intestinal parasitic infestations or infections.

Methods of treatment:
We use leaf juice and bitters of Aloe ferox as main treatment or as supplementary treatment or as prophylactic treatment after keen observation and anticipation of severity of toxicity, severity of imbalance and strength of patient.

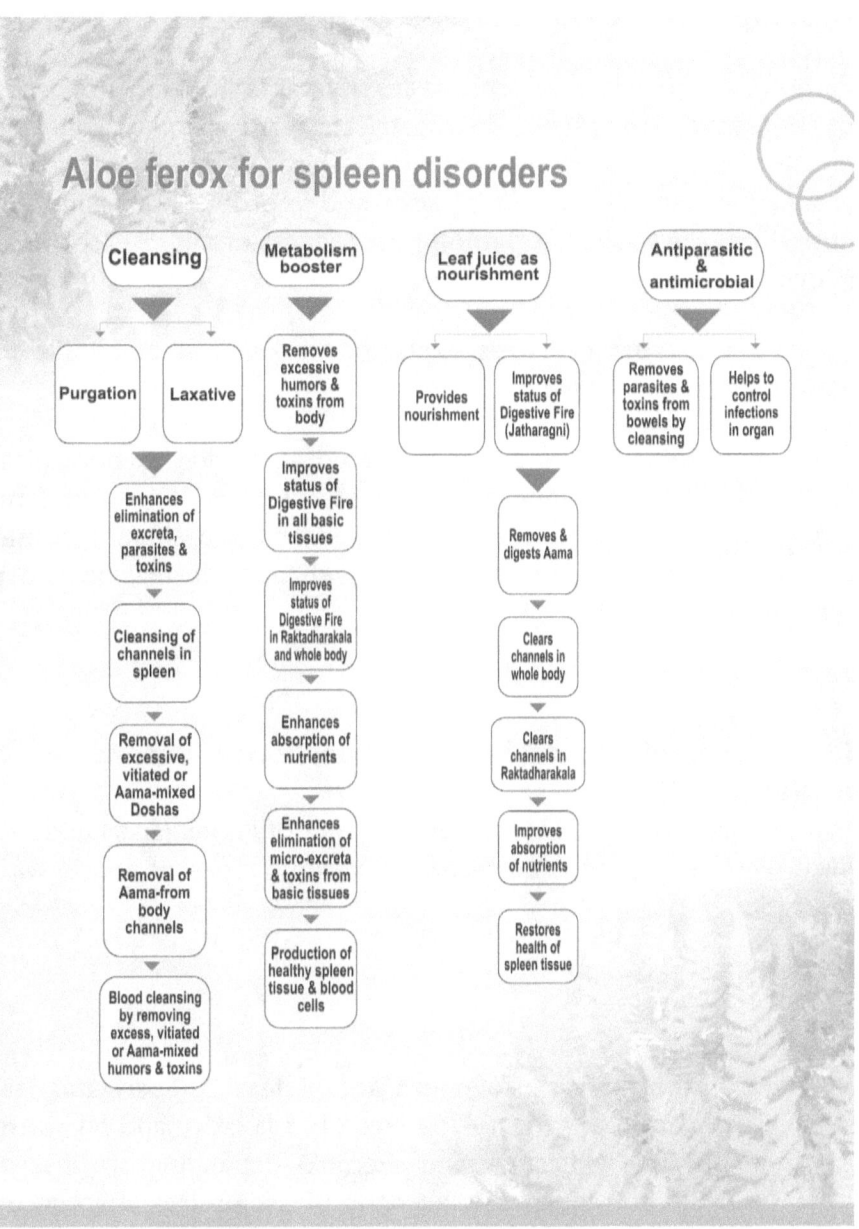

Aloe ferox for spleen disorders

Cleansing

Purgation | Laxative

Enhances elimination of excreta, parasites & toxins

Cleansing of channels in spleen

Removal of excessive, vitiated or Aama-mixed Doshas

Removal of Aama-from body channels

Blood cleansing by removing excess, vitiated or Aama-mixed humors & toxins

Metabolism booster

Removes excessive humors & toxins from body

Improves status of Digestive Fire in all basic tissues

Improves status of Digestive Fire in Raktadharakala and whole body

Enhances absorption of nutrients

Enhances elimination of micro-excreta & toxins from basic tissues

Production of healthy spleen tissue & blood cells

Leaf juice as nourishment

Provides nourishment | Improves status of Digestive Fire (Jatharagni)

Removes & digests Aama

Clears channels in whole body

Clears channels in Raktadharakala

Improves absorption of nutrients

Restores health of spleen tissue

Antiparasitic & antimicrobial

Removes parasites & toxins from bowels by cleansing | Helps to control infections in organ

Aloe ferox for ascitis

Concept of ascitis in short according to *Ayurveda*
Ascitis is named as '*Udar*' in *Ayurvedic* Texts.

Pathological process of this disease starts from disturbance of 'Digestive Fire' (*Agni*). This leads to aggravation of *Vata* and production of '*Aaam*' at the same time. This leads to obstruction of channels in various systems of body and improper assimilation of nutrients. Due to specific pathological process of this disease, fluids get collected in peritoneal cavity.

There are 8 types of ascitis explained in *Ayurvedic* texts due to various causes.

Though these various types are treated according to etiological factors, line of treatment includes restoration of 'Digestive Fire' (*Agni*), improving micro-digestion of food or the basic metabolism on cellular level and removing the toxins through normal excretory system.

Pharmacological actions of Aloe ferox according to *Ayurveda*:
We can use exudate (*Niryas*), solid extract of leaves (*Saar*) and leaf juice (*Patraswaras*) of Aloe ferox for various types of ascitis with discretion.

It can help in following ways:

1. Cleansing –
- Exudate (*Niryas*), solid extract of leaves (*Saar*) and leaf juice (*Patraswaras*) of Aloe ferox has laxative and purgative properties (*anulomak* and *virechak*) depending on dosage. Alongwith vigorous treatment of ascitis like *virechan* or tapping of collected fluid in modern medicine, we can use Aloe ferox in any form depending on severity of symptoms, accumulation of toxins and strength of patient.

- It will help to remove toxins along with feaces and the remaining fluid.

- This will help to remove aggravated and vitiated *Doshas* in all types explained by *Ayurveda* with discretion.

- For *Chidrodar* (type of ascitis due to puncture of intestines), we have to use Aloe ferox as prophylactic.

2. Restoration of 'Digestive Fire' (*Jatharagni*) and improvement of basic metabolism at cellular level (*Dhatvagnivardhan*) –

Aloe ferox can improve main 'Digestive Fire' and other 12 'Digestive Fire' too (seven types for basic tissues or *Dhatu*s and five types for components made of five universal elements). This leads to improved appetite, digestion, assimilation and can also act as booster for basic metabolism on cellular level. This helps to improve general health and immunity in patients.

3. As a tonic for organs involved in pathological process of Ascitis –

Aloe ferox can work as anti-inflammatory (*Shothaghna*) and excellent tonic for improving functions of organs like liver, spleen, pancreas, intestines and channels of system controlling metabolism of liquid part of diet (*Udakvahasrotas*). It will remove obstruction in channels (*Srotorodha*) and also as booster for metabolism of those systems. This can be used as supplement for treatment of all types of ascitis and also as prophylactic treatment.

4. Nutritional supplement –

Aloe ferox can help in two ways as nutritional supplement:

- Nutrients in leaf sap of Aloe ferox can help patients to get good nourishment.

- It can act as booster for better absorption and metabolism of food.

5. Anti-parasitic and Anti-microbial treatment – Aloe ferox can help as antimicrobial and antiparasitic (*Kruminashak*) according to *Ayurveda*.

Methods of treatment:
We can use Aloe ferox as part of main treatment, as supportive treatment and even as prophylactic treatment as per requirements.

We can use exudates and leaf extract (Aloe Bitters) for cleansing, as metabolism booster and tonic for *Udakavahasrotas* and other organs involved in pathology, in small doses frequently with discretion.

Leaf juice of Aloe ferox can be used internally as nutritional supplement and also as prophylactic treatment till we get signs of improvement in *Udakavahasrotas* and general health.

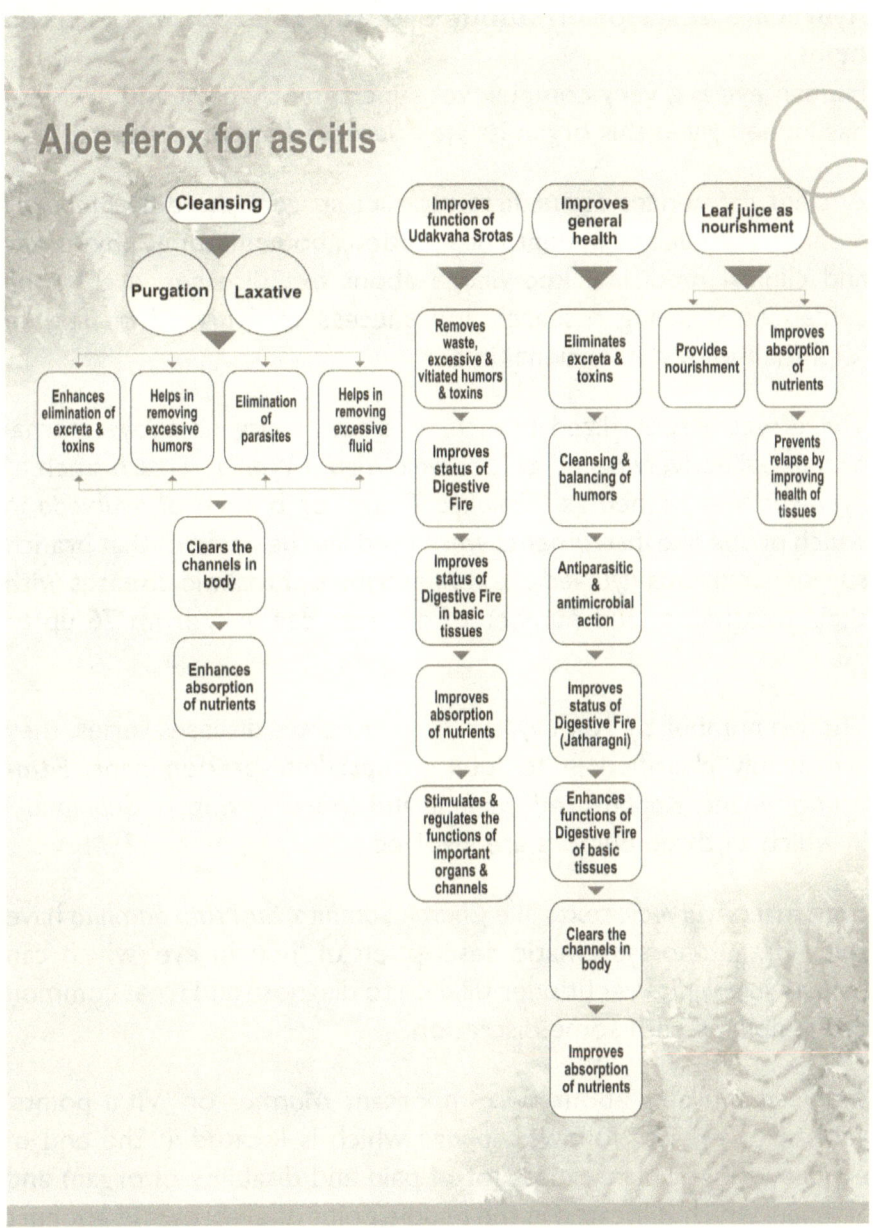

Aloe ferox for ascitis

Cleansing

Purgation | Laxative

- Enhances elimination of excreta & toxins
- Helps in removing excessive humors
- Elimination of parasites
- Helps in removing excessive fluid

Clears the channels in body

Enhances absorption of nutrients

Improves function of Udakvaha Srotas

Removes waste, excessive & vitiated humors & toxins

Improves status of Digestive Fire

Improves status of Digestive Fire in basic tissues

Improves absorption of nutrients

Stimulates & regulates the functions of important organs & channels

Improves general health

Eliminates excreta & toxins

Cleansing & balancing of humors

Antiparasitic & antimicrobial action

Improves status of Digestive Fire (Jatharagni)

Enhances functions of Digestive Fire of basic tissues

Clears the channels in body

Improves absorption of nutrients

Leaf juice as nourishment

Provides nourishment

Improves absorption of nutrients

Prevents relapse by improving health of tissues

Aloe ferox for ophthalmological problems (diseases of eyes)

Ayurvedic description about eye and related problems in brief

Human eye is a very complex yet superb mechanism and *Ayurveda* has indeed given this organ its well-deserved importance.

Ancient references about first cataract surgery done by *Maharshi Sushruta* in India and in depth description about anatomy, physiology and clinical medicinal knowledge about eye diseases, are strong evidences showing research and success of *Ayurveda* in field of 'Ophthalmology' in ancient times.

There was a specialized branch to treat all organs above sternal notch, collectively called as '*Urdhvajatrugata Vyadhi*'. That branch of *Ayurveda* was named as '*Shalakya Tantra*' or branch of *Ayurveda* in which probe like instruments were used, as the name of that branch suggests. Various *Ayurvedic* texts describe ophthalmic diseases with their treatments and number of diseases can vary from 76 up to 96.

Though number of '*Netravyadhi*' or ophthalmic diseases varies, they are mainly classified in to four groups: *Vata*-predominant, *Pitta*-predominant, *Kapha*-predominant and fourth group is '*Sannipatik*' in which all three humors are involved.

Even main *Ayurvedic* texts like *Charak Samhita, Sushruta Samhita* have given detail and systematic description of 'human eye' which can help an *Ayurvedic* Practitioner till date to diagnose and treat common eye problems with some discretion.

Ayurveda explains about two important *Marmas* or 'Vital points' related to eyes as follows; *Apanga* which is located at the end of eyebrow (if got hurt causes lot of pain and disability of organ) and *Sthapani* which is located in the middle point of eyebrows (if got hurt can cause immediate death).

Though treatments also include surgical procedures, there are some interesting cleansing methods and alleviation treatments mentioned as *Anjan, Netratarpan, Putpak, Aschotan* etc.

Pharmacological actions of Aloe ferox according to *Ayurveda*:

Eye diseases can be treated internally and externally with the help of Aloe ferox.

Internal treatment:

When ophthalmic diseases occur due to imbalance in all over body or as side-effects then, Aloe ferox can be used internally.

We can use it as main treatment or supplementary treatment as follows:

I. Cleansing –

- **Purgation of accumulated excreta, parasites and toxins from body through bowels** – Due to purgative properties, Aloe Bitters can be used for thorough cleansing with proper care. This will help to remove all the excreta, toxins and parasites from bowels.

- **Cleansing of body channels** – Aloe ferox can help for cleansing the micro-channels in body.

- **Removal of excessive and *Aama*-mixed or toxin-mixed humors** – If there are associated digestive disorders due to aggravation or vitiation of humors especially due to *Aama*, mild laxative properties of Aloe ferox can be used for a prolonged period. This action will also help for slow but constant removal of excessive, vitiated or *Aama*-mixed humors along with excreta and toxins produced due to imbalance in quantity and functions of humors. If there are symptoms due to vitiation of blood because of excessive, vitiated or *Aama*-mixed humors especially *Pitta*, then considering the relation of *Pitta* humor with blood, we can use Aloe ferox for mild laxative action which will help in related types of symptoms.

- **Cleansing of blood** – When certain ophthalmological problems include vitiation of blood, blood cleansing action of Aloe ferox can be a major part of treatment. We can use mild laxative action of Aloe ferox in symptoms occurring due to malfunction or vitiation of blood. This action will help for slow but constant removal of excessive, vitiated or *Aama*-mixed humors especially *Pitta* from blood which will ultimately help to cure infections and will also restore functions of main internal organs.

Cleansing action with all above aspects can be helpful for fast recovery.

2. Metabolism booster –

Taste (*Rasa*), Postdigestive effect (*Vipak*) and Active energy (*Veerya*) along with its properties (*Gunas*) can help as effective medicine to boost functions of 13 types of 'Digestive Fire' in body. Though there are 13 types, other 12 types are dependent on main entity which is *Jatharagni* or 'Digestive Fire' situated in stomach, duodenum and pancreatic area.

Normal functions of this type of 'Digestive Fire' depend on status of *Pitta* humor in body.

Aloe ferox helps to cleanse the micro and macro-channels in body, removes root cause of all imbalances which can be excessive and impure humors. It can be good activator for organs like liver, gall bladder and intestines to secret more digestive juices.

It can help to restore the functions of 'Digestive Fire' as well, which allover help to improve appetite, digestion and assimilation of nutrients. This can also help as general health booster and immunity booster by improving the cellular level metabolism in body.

3. Maintaining the balance of humors –

Cleansing action removes excessive and vitiated humors while qualities like *Rasa, Veerya, Vipak* as explained in chapter No. 4 help in balancing the humors if required further.

Removal of vitiated and excessive *Vata* along with *Vata* alleviating qualities of Aloe ferox will help to reduce *Vata* - related symptoms like sharp pain, lack of muscle control etc.

Removal of vitiated and excessive *Pitta* along with *Pitta* alleviating qualities of Aloe ferox will help to reduce *Pitta* - related symptoms like inflammation, burning sensation etc.

Removal of vitiated and excessive *Kapha* along with *Kapha* alleviating qualities of Aloe ferox will help to reduce *Kapha* - related symptoms like swelling, heaviness etc.

4. Nourishment of *Dhatu* –

In conditions showing malnourishment and loss of weight, we can use Aloe ferox as nutritional supplement for restoration of quantity and functions of basic tissues (*Dhatu*). All actions of this plant can help to improve absorption and assimilation of nutrients in all seven basic tissues (*Dhatu*) the order and will also help for healing our body inside out.

Nutritional qualities of leaf pulp of Aloe ferox can help directly as supplement.

5. Antiparasitic and antimicrobial action –

Aloe ferox can show action as anti-parasitic (*krumighna*) and as anti-microbial which can be used for treatment of intestinal parasitic infestations or infections.

External treatment –

It can also be used as external treatment in various forms of treatments given in *Ayurvedic* texts.

It can provide a soothing, cool and anti-microbial application which will be a good local treatment in symptoms like redness of eyes, secretions, burning sensation and pain of eyes.

Methods of treatment:
Leaf juice can be used as *Anjan* by applying aloe juice like *Kajal* or as *Aschotan* or eye drops.

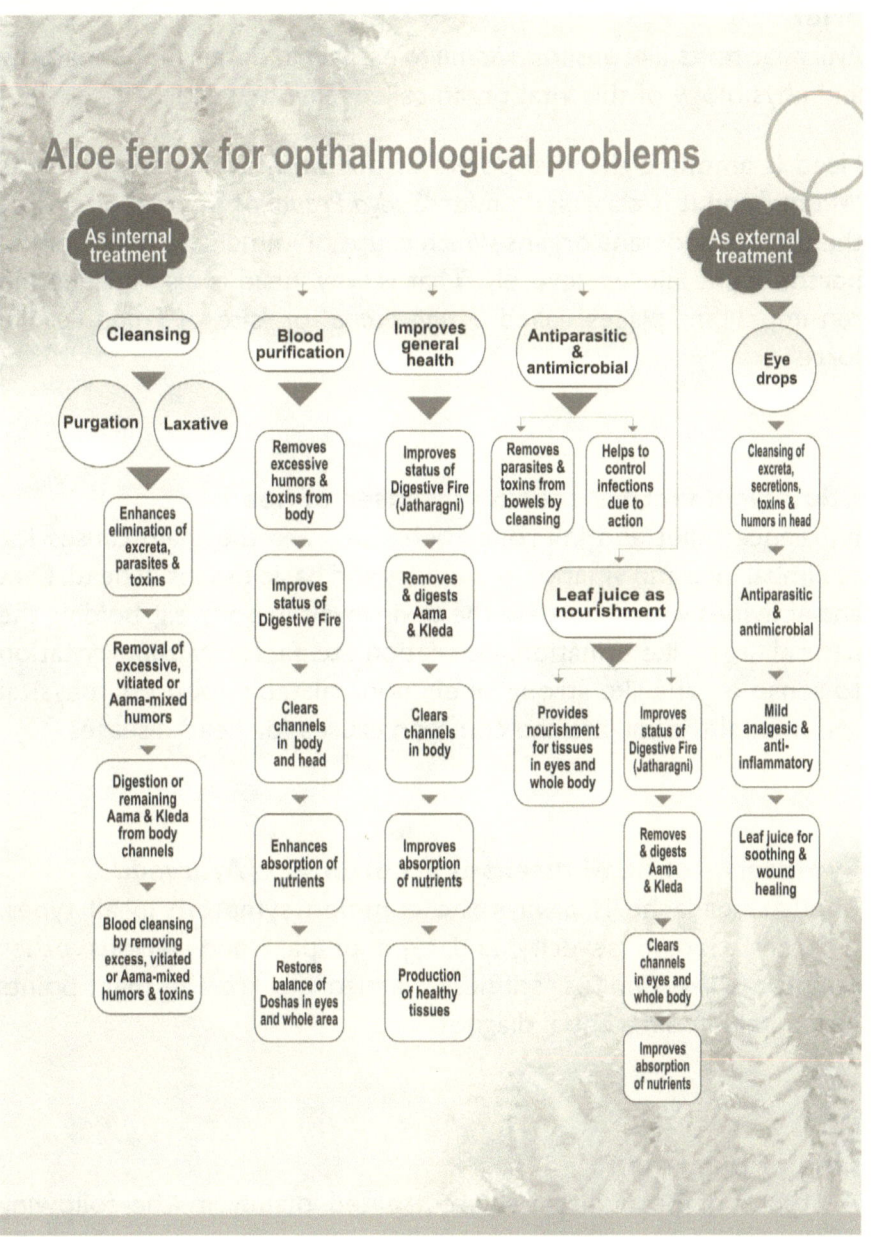

Aloe ferox for opthalmological problems

As internal treatment

As external treatment

| Cleansing | Blood purification | Improves general health | Antiparasitic & antimicrobial | | Eye drops |

Purgation | **Laxative**

Enhances elimination of excreta, parasites & toxins

Removes excessive humors & toxins from body

Improves status of Digestive Fire (Jatharagni)

Removes parasites & toxins from bowels by cleansing

Helps to control infections due to action

Cleansing of excreta, secretions, toxins & humors in head

Removal of excessive, vitiated or Aama-mixed humors

Improves status of Digestive Fire

Removes & digests Aama & Kleda

Leaf juice as nourishment

Antiparasitic & antimicrobial

Digestion or remaining Aama & Kleda from body channels

Clears channels in body and head

Clears channels in body

Provides nourishment for tissues in eyes and whole body

Improves status of Digestive Fire (Jatharagni)

Mild analgesic & anti-inflammatory

Blood cleansing by removing excess, vitiated or Aama-mixed humors & toxins

Enhances absorption of nutrients

Improves absorption of nutrients

Removes & digests Aama & Kleda

Leaf juice for soothing & wound healing

Restores balance of Doshas in eyes and whole area

Production of healthy tissues

Clears channels in eyes and whole body

Improves absorption of nutrients

Aloe ferox in headaches

Ayurvedic concept and patho-physiology of headache in brief

Ayurvedic texts like *Sushruta Samhita* explain in detail about anatomy and physiology of this vital organ called '*Shir*' or head.

Head is among eight vital points of our body which are called as '*Marma*' and it is classified under '*Sadya Pranahar Marma*' or one of the those important organs which cause of immediate death of the person if get injured severely. That is why, head is also included in ten important places called '*Pranayatana*' or 'site of *Prana* i.e. life force'.

Etiological factors causing diseases of head

Imbalanced diet and improper behaviour are the main causes for the imbalance and vitiation of humors and basic tissues in head. Diet and activities which increase the toxin levels in body e.g. holding the natural urges like urination, defecation etc, factor causing irritation to sense organs like strong smell, non-palatable food etc, physical and mental trauma are the common causes for head diseases.

Symptoms of head diseases according to *Ayurveda*

Though headache is always the common symptom in all types, differentiation in severity and type of pain and various other symptoms like tinnitus, stiffness, vertigo etc are the main points which help in differential diagnosis.

Line of treatment

All types of head diseases are treated mainly in the following sequence:

1. Cleansing (where applicable) –
Various types of herbs are used to remove the aggravated or vitiated *Doshas* from head by using various methods in *panchakarma* like *Shirovirechan, Dhoompaan, Shirobasti* etc.

2. Alleviation –
Remaining amount of humors is alleviated with the help of herbs having antagonist properties to that humor.

3. Nourishment –
Humors (*Dosha*) and basic tissues (*Dhatu*) which are less in quantity are replenished by using herbs having similar properties.

Ayurvedic types of diseases of head
Ancient *Ayurvedic* text called *Charak Samhita* has mentioned about five types of diseases of head called *Shiroroga* on the basis of etiological factors as follows:

Vataj – *Vata*-predominant

Pittaj – *Pitta*-predominant

Kaphaj – *Kapha*-predominant

Sannipatik – all three humors involved

Krumij – caused due to microorganisms

Another important text called *Sushruta Samhita* has added two more types as follows:

Raktaj – caused by toxins in blood

Kshayaj – caused by depleted humors and basic tissues in head

Allover there are eleven types mentioned in *Sushruta Samhita*.

Pharmacological actions of Aloe ferox according to *Ayurveda*:

We can use Aloe ferox for various head diseases (*Shiroroga*) after accurate diagnosis with thorough examination.

In case of headache associated with other symptoms due to some systemic disease and headache as main symptom due to diseases of head mentioned according to *Ayurveda*, we can use this plant as internal treatment; oral or nasal.

We can use it as main treatment or supplementary treatment as well.

Internal treatment:

As a part of internal treatment for oral use, this plant will show following actions:

1. Cleansing –

- **Purgation of accumulated excreta, parasites and toxins from body through bowels** – Due to purgative properties, Aloe Bitters can be used for thorough cleansing with proper care. This will help to remove all the excreta, toxins and parasites from bowels.

- **Cleansing of body channels** – Aloe ferox can help for cleansing the micro-channels in body.

- **Removal of excessive and *Aama*-mixed or toxin-mixed humors** – If symptoms are due to aggravation or vitiation of humors especially due to *Aama*, mild laxative properties of Aloe ferox can be used for a prolonged period. This action will also help for slow but constant removal of excessive, vitiated or *Aama*-mixed humors along with excreta and toxins produced due to imbalance in quantity and functions of humors. If there are symptoms due to vitiation of blood because of excessive, vitiated or *Aama*-mixed humors especially *Pitta*, then considering the relation of *Pitta* humor with blood, we can use Aloe ferox for mild laxative action which will help in related types of symptoms.

- **Cleansing of blood** – When head diseases are caused by vitiation of blood i.e. *Pittaj, Raktaj* and *Krumij*, blood cleansing action of Aloe ferox can be a major part of treatment. We can use mild laxative action of Aloe ferox in symptoms occurring due to malfunction or vitiation of blood. This action will help for slow but constant removal of excessive, vitiated or *Aama*-mixed humors especially *Pitta* from blood which will ultimately help to cure infections and will also restore functions of main internal organs.

Cleansing action with all above aspects can be helpful for fast recovery from the head problems due to systemic or local problems.

2. Metabolism booster –
Taste (*Rasa*), Postdigestive effect (*Vipak*) and Active energy (*Veerya*) along with its properties (*Gunas*) can help as effective medicine to boost functions of 13 types of 'Digestive Fire' in body. Though there are 13 types, other 12 types are dependent on main entity which is *Jatharagni* or 'Digestive Fire' situated in stomach, duodenum and pancreatic area.

Normal functions of this type of 'Digestive Fire' depend on status of *Pitta* humor in body.

Aloe ferox helps to cleanse the micro and macro-channels in body, removes root cause of all imbalances which can be excessive and impure humors. It can be good activator for organs like liver, gall bladder and intestines to secret more digestive juices.

It can help to restore the functions of 'Digestive Fire' and allover helps to improve appetite, digestion and assimilation of nutrients.

This can also help as general health booster and immunity booster by improving the cellular level metabolism in body.

When head diseases are due to systemic problems having lowered Digestive Fire, then this action will help.

3. Maintaining of balance of humors –
Cleansing action removes excessive and vitiated humors while qualities like *Rasa, Veerya, Vipak* as explained in chapter No. 4 help in balancing the humors if required further.

Removal of vitiated and excessive *Vata* along with *Vata* alleviating qualities of Aloe ferox will help to reduce *Vata* - related symptoms like sharp pain, stiffness, tinnitus etc.

Removal of vitiated and excessive *Pitta* along with *Pitta* alleviating qualities of Aloe ferox will help to reduce *Pitta* - related symptoms like burning sensation, fever, inflammation etc.

Removal of vitiated and excessive *Kapha* along with *Kapha* alleviating qualities of Aloe ferox will help to reduce *Kapha* - related symptoms like swelling, heaviness etc.

4. Nourishment of *Dhatu* –
In conditions showing malnourishment and loss of weight, we can use Aloe ferox as nutritional supplement for restoration of quantity and functions of all the seven types of basic tissues (*Dhatu*). All actions of this plant can help to improve absorption and assimilation of nutrients in all *Dhatu* (seven basic types of tissues) in the order and will also help for healing our body inside out.

Nutritional qualities of leaf pulp of Aloe ferox can help directly as supplement.

This action can also help in *Kshayaj* type.

5. Antiparasitic and antimicrobial action –
Aloe ferox can show action as anti-parasitic (*krumighna*) and as anti-microbial which can be used to treat intestinal parasitic infestations

or infections. This can help in systemic causes of headache and also in headache due to infective type called *Krumij*.

Nasal treatment –

The same actions can help in treatments given by nasal route.

External treatment –

It can also be used as external treatment in various forms of treatments given in *Ayurvedic* texts.

It can provide a soothing, cool and anti-microbial application which will be a good local treatment in headaches with swelling e.g. headache due to trauma or in sinusitis etc.

Methods of treatment:

We can use Cape Aloe or Aloe Bitters in very less dose like 100-300mg, depending upon general strength and severity of ailment, as oral administration.

We can also include traces of Cape Aloe or Aloe Bitters as nasal treatment in *Panchakarma* called *Shirovirechan*.

We can supplement Aloe ferox with some anti-inflammatory and analgesic herbs as part of headaches or other symptoms due to head diseases associated to systemic diseases.

We can use Cape Aloe or boiled and dried leaf juice of Aloe ferox in very less dose as part of internal or local treatment where cleansing, metabolism boost and improvement in general health is required.

In conditions having general weakness, anemia and other debilitating diseases that require nourishment, leaf juice can be used orally in dosage from 10 ml to 30 ml as per strength of patient and severity of symptoms, as part of nourishment. We can use leaf juice of Aloe ferox.

We can use leaf sap as local application on forehead and scalp to reduce headache.

In conditions that require local soothing or healing properties, leaf juice can be administered in nose which will act as local anti-inflammatory, mild analgesic, tonic and anti-septic herb e.g. in migraine and sinusitis.

Caution:
Aloe ferox should be avoided in pregnant women as its use can cause abortions.

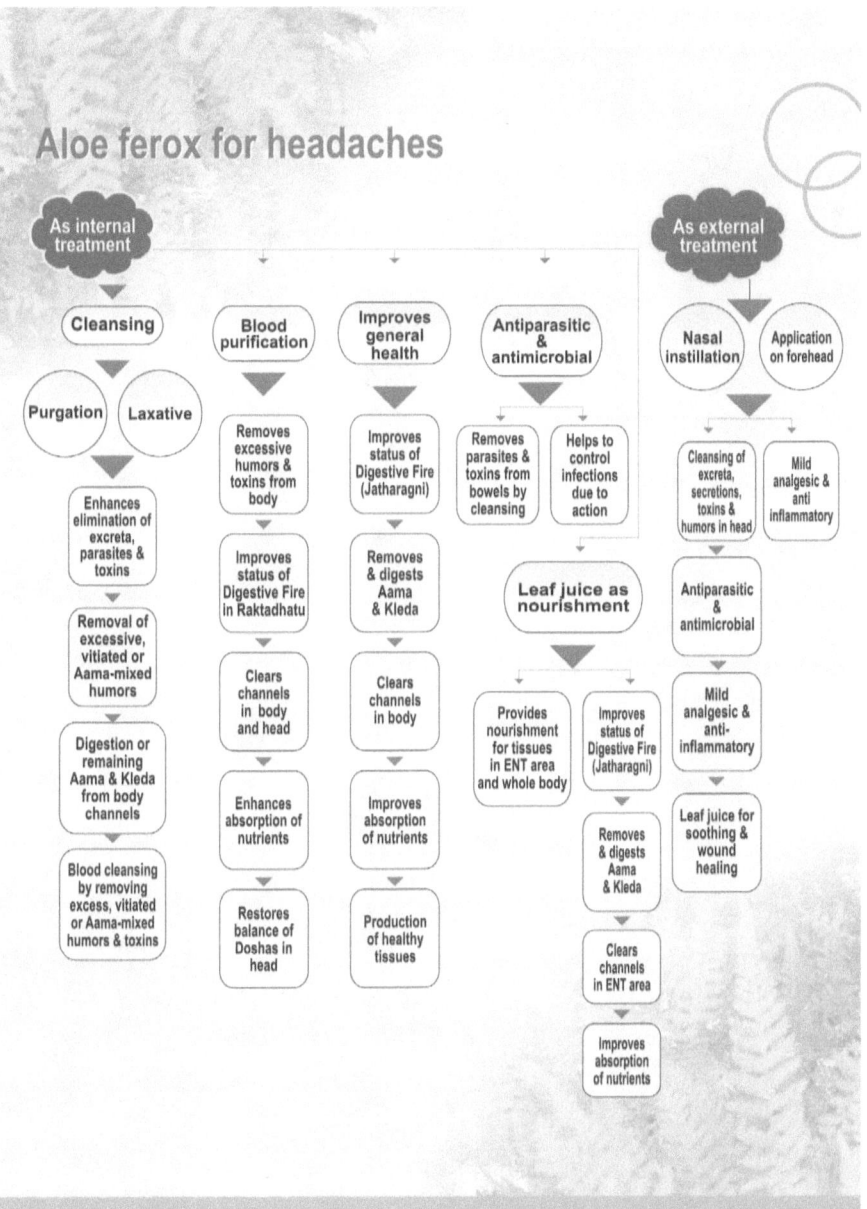

Aloe ferox for headaches

As internal treatment

Cleansing

Purgation | Laxative

Enhances elimination of excreta, parasites & toxins

Removal of excessive, vitiated or Aama-mixed humors

Digestion or remaining Aama & Kleda from body channels

Blood cleansing by removing excess, vitiated or Aama-mixed humors & toxins

Blood purification

Removes excessive humors & toxins from body

Improves status of Digestive Fire in Raktadhatu

Clears channels in body and head

Enhances absorption of nutrients

Restores balance of Doshas in head

Improves general health

Improves status of Digestive Fire (Jatharagni)

Removes & digests Aama & Kleda

Clears channels in body

Improves absorption of nutrients

Production of healthy tissues

Antiparasitic & antimicrobial

Removes parasites & toxins from bowels by cleansing

Helps to control infections due to action

Leaf juice as nourishment

Provides nourishment for tissues in ENT area and whole body

Improves status of Digestive Fire (Jatharagni)

Removes & digests Aama & Kleda

Clears channels in ENT area

Improves absorption of nutrients

As external treatment

Nasal instillation | Application on forehead

Cleansing of excreta, secretions, toxins & humors in head

Mild analgesic & anti inflammatory

Antiparasitic & antimicrobial

Mild analgesic & anti-inflammatory

Leaf juice for soothing & wound healing

131

REFERENCES

1. *Ayurvedic* Philosophy; Author- Prof. P. H. Kulkarni

2. *Kaya-Chikitsa*; Author- Dr. Y. G. Joshi

3. *Marathi Sushruta Samhita* - Part 1, 2, 3; Translated by - Prof. P. H. Kulkarni

4. *Marathi Charak Samhita* - Part 1, 2; Translated by - Prof. P. H. Kulkarni

ACKNOWLEDGEMENT

I am eternally thankful to my family members and my Guru, Prof. P. H. Kulkarni for their support, efforts, blessings and many many more things they ever did for me.

My heartfelt gratitude is also due to the whole team of AutherHouse Publications.

My thanks are also due to Mr. Gajanan More, team member of 'Kesari', for graphic designing.

Special Thanks to 'House of Aloes' for allowing us to use images of various beautiful specimen of Aloe ferox.

Website used for images of Aloe ferox from various places of South Africa:

www.southafrica.info

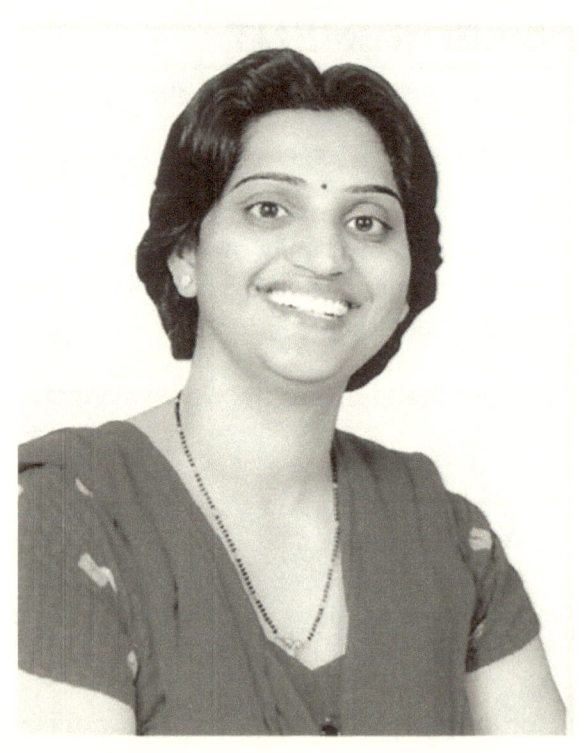

ABOUT THE AUTHOR

Dr. Sharduli is an Ayurvedic Doctor working in South Africa and India as well.

Education:
- Bachelor of Ayurvedic Medicine and Surgery - B.A.M.S , Shivaji University, India
- Fellowship from Institute of Indian Medicine, India.
- Ayurveda Parangat (Doctor of Ayurveda), European Ayurveda Academy, Italy
- Ayurveda Varidhi (Doctorate in Ayurveda) ,European Ayurveda Academy, Italy

Awards:
- Vanamitra Puraskar', Vaidya Khadiwale Research Institute, Pune, India.
- 'Dr. J. D. Apte National Award for excellent work in research of medicinal plants', Warana Research Trust, Sangli, India.
- 'Young Scientist Award' , Australasian Academy of Ayurveda and Yoga, Sydney, Australia
- 'Award for international excellence in field of Ayurveda', Panacea International Conference on Ayurveda and Yoga, Mauritius.

- 'International Award for women' by 'Deerghayu International' in category of NRI women working for promotion and propagation of Ayurveda'

Literary work:
- Number of research papers, articles and reviews on Ayurveda published in research journals of complimentary medicine and journals of Ayurveda in India, Italy, Australia, South Africa and also on Internet Journals.
- General articles are published in health magazines like Odyssey, Health Encounters, Healer etc.
- Her general articles showing various aspects of South Africa, written in her regional language, Marathi, are published in Indian Newspapers.

Books:
- Medicinal Plants of South Africa – In Ayurvedic point of view
- Enjoy seasons in South Africa – with Ayurveda
- Think before you drink water
- South Africa – Ek Indradhanushi desh (South Africa – a rainbow nation) (Marathi Language)

Designations:
- Founder CEO, The Ayurveda Foundation – South Africa (TAFSA), Johannesburg, South Africa
- Co-ordinator, Ayurveda Faculty, Sangli Campus, Tilak Maharashtra University, India
- Advisor and active committee member for Certificate course of Natural Medicine, Wits University, South Africa
- Ayurveda Facilitator, Traditional Healers' Organization, South Africa
- Global Advisor, BHHAS, India
- Member of Editorial team of Healer Magazine, South Africa and Deerghayu International, India

www.ingramcontent.com/pod-product-compliance
Lightning Source LLC
Chambersburg PA
CBHW020441290526
45785CB00002B/959